Joint Education and Training Library

This book is to be returned on or before the last date stamped below. Overdue charges will be incurred by the late return of books.

Renew in person, by phone (01270 612538, or internal x2538/3172) or online at: http://libcat.chester.ac.uk (NHS staff ask for password)

A Beginner's Guide to Evidence-Based Practice in Health and Social Care

Third Edition

Helen Aveyard and Pam Sharp

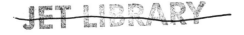

Open University Press

Open University Press
McGraw-Hill Education
8th Floor, 338 Euston Road
London
England
NW1 3BH

email: enquiries@openup.co.uk
world wide web: www.openup.co.uk

and Two Penn Plaza, New York, NY 10121-2289, USA

First edition published 2009
Second edition published 2013
Published in this 3rd Edition 2017

A catalogue record of this book is available from the British Library

ISBN-13: 978-0-335-22708-2
ISBN-10: 0-33-522708-2
eISBN: 978-0-335-22709-9

Library of Congress Cataloging-in-Publication Data
CIP data applied for

Typeset by Transforma Pvt. Ltd., Chennai, India

Printed in Great Britain by Bell and Bain Ltd, Glasgow

Fictitious names of companies, products, people, characters and/or data that may be used herein (in case studies or in examples) are not intended to represent any real individual, company, product or event.

Praise for this book

"This highly engaging book is a 'must-have' for health professionals who want to navigate their way through the professional and scientific literature and find the best available evidence to inform their decision-making."

Debra Jackson, Professor of Nursing,
Oxford Brookes University, UK and
University of Technology,
Sydney (UTS), Australia

"This 3rd edition is an ideal text for undergraduate and post-graduate students as well as clinicians wanting to extend their practice in an evidence-based manner. It is presented in an engaging style that draws the reader in and the language is pitched to inform and educate a broad audience. A diverse range of examples are included to highlight key points so as to appeal to readers from a range of backgrounds. Overall this is a must-have text for a wide audience."

Professor Elizabeth Halcomb,
Professor of Primary Health Care Nursing,
University of Wollongong, Australia

Contents

6   How do I know if the evidence is convincing and useful?   137

7   How to implement evidence-based practice   176

Acknowledgements

Pam Sharp would like to thank Tim Sharp for his ongoing love and support and to Elaine Bethell, a nurse and friend for many years.

Helen Aveyard would like to thank the Aveyard and Gregory family for their love and support.

Introduction

This book is for you if you are:

- A student starting out or undertaking a pre-registration course in any of the health and social care professions.
- A registered practitioner returning to post-qualification study or to practice after a career break.
- Anyone who feels clinically or professionally 'out of date' or has ever said, '*I am not an academic . . . I am practical*' or '*I've always done it this way*'.
- A practice assessor/mentor[1] who is supporting students in practice and aware of the need to use evidence in your daily practice and to role-model best practice to your students.

This book is also for you if you know that:

- You are legally and professionally accountable for your practice once you are a registered practitioner.
- As a student you may be called to account by your university or institution of higher education.
- There is a large amount and many different types of information available.
- Skills are required to find, understand, and use information.
- In order to practise safely and/or to be successful as a student (pre- or post-qualifying) or member of staff, you need to know how to apply relevant information to your practice and in your written work.

So . . . where do you start?

You may feel that you do not know where to begin to use this evidence in your practice and learning or that when you try to, it is too complicated or

---

1 The term practice assessor/mentor will be used throughout to describe those who support learners in practice. A variety of terms are used throughout the professions such as: clinical educator, supervisor, practice educator/teacher, clinical tutor or instructor.

difficult. This book will lead you through this process at an introductory level in a jargon-free way.

Aim of this book

The aim of this book is to explain evidence-based practice (EBP) and to present it as a topic that practitioners at all levels, including students, can relate to from the very start of their professional experience and in their writing. Evidence-based practice is of course a practical topic; however, we are aware that it is assessed in academic writing and is a major component in almost all marking criteria for those studying for a professional qualification in health and social care.

A Beginner's Guide to Evidence-Based Practice in Health and Social Care provides a step-by-step approach to using evidence in practice in a practical and straightforward way.

Examples

In this revised edition, we have included examples that may be understood by a range of professionals in a range of contexts, both nationally and internationally, as we all work within a wider team. We would ask that you read through the examples even if they may not relate directly to your specialty and think broadly about the message the example is giving.

How to get the most from this book

- It is best if you read the introductory chapters first, as the book is presented in the order in which we think it should be read, but you can use the index if you have a particular issue you want to find out about.
- Use the glossary for explanations of words you are unfamiliar with.
- Work with a colleague or a student who is more confident in using evidence in practice.
- Access the Internet and start practising your search skills using relevant databases (don't leave it until you really need to find information quickly).
- Do some additional reading around the topic of evidence-based practice.
- Contact your local health and social care librarian (through your work organization or local university) for additional, practical training

sessions. Some university libraries have specialist health and social care librarians.
- Don't give up if you find something difficult or don't understand it. Feel good about every new thing that you have learnt.

The symbols used in this book

Key information

Think point

Activity for you to do

Key web link

1 What is evidence-based practice?

- Defining evidence-based practice
- Exploring the components of evidence-based practice
- Consequences of not taking an evidence-based approach
- What does evidence-based practice mean to me?
- In summary
- Key points
- Quiz questions

 Put simply, evidence-based practice (EBP) is practice that is supported by the best available evidence, taking into account the patient's/client's preferences and using your own judgement. If we practise an evidence-based approach, then we are set to give the best possible care.

Sounds complicated? It's not really, just read on . . .

Evidence-based practice starts with the following principle:

Have evidence-informed reasons for your practice decisions and the care provided

If you are a **student** starting out on a course in any of the health and social care professions, you are likely to be well aware of the need to be able to explain the care that you give both in practice and in the assignments you write. This is because patients and clients expect you, even as a student, to understand why you are caring for them in a particular way and to explain the reasons (which should usually be based on the best available evidence) for the care you provide. This becomes increasingly important as you gain experience and become the one who is planning care and making decisions relating to care, rather than acting in a more supportive role. In fact, being able to explain a good rationale for practice decisions and planning care is something that distinguishes registered health and social care practitioners from others in the wide variety of assistant and supporting roles.

If you are a **registered practitioner**, you may feel that you cannot always give a thorough rationale for your practice, and fear that your practice may not be as up-to-date as it could be, which can make you feel vulnerable or under-confident. You may not have been able to access professional development opportunities, or you may be about to re-commence your studies and want to find out how to use evidence in your academic work. You may increasingly be delegating care delivery to others and you need to be able to justify what you are asking others to do.

If you are a **practice assessor/mentor** supervising learners or a **practitioner** who is returning to work or study after a career break, you are likely to be even more aware of this need. You may feel you lack the skills to act as a role model for best practice and lack confidence in giving reasons for your practice to others.

A vital part of evidence-based practice is being able to explain the care that you give. In most cases, this involves referring to the best available evidence. Consider the following examples:

Examples from practice

Example 1: Imagine you are a social work student. Your current placement is with a multidisciplinary team that works in a deprived area of the country. The caseload includes a lot of disadvantaged families. You visit one family in which one of the children, a 5-year-old boy, has behavioural problems. The family are given advice about attending a parenting skills programme for help in managing the behaviour of the child. When you leave the family home, you ask your practice assessor/mentor why this has been advised. They explain that recent research evidence has indicated that support provided by parenting groups can help parents to manage the behaviour of their child and to relieve their own stress and anxiety caused by the child's difficulties (Barlow 2016).

Example 2: Imagine you are a mental health or social work student working with people who are recovering from depression. Your mentor advises you about the importance of close follow-up with clients because of the risk of suicide among this population. Your mentor explains that research undertaken by Appleby et al. in 1999 has demonstrated the importance of follow-up and that supporting individuals recovering from a mental health issue has been shown to decrease their suicide risk.

The above two examples demonstrate a practitioner using an evidence-based approach. Now consider the third example:

Example 3: Imagine you are working in a travel vaccination clinic and are consulted by a patient who is travelling far afield on a gap year. The patient asks you in a lot of detail for information about the risks and benefits of various vaccinations and you do not feel confident to answer her questions. In fact, some of her questions remind you that you are not as fully aware of the rationale for the advice given as you might be. You resort to statements such as, 'This is what we always give to people going to that area . . .' but you can sense that the patient is keen to know more to ensure that she is fully protected and to consider any alternative courses of action that might be available to her, including altering her travel plans. You end the consultation feeling that you have not provided evidence-based advice.

You will see from these simple examples that as a student or registered member of staff, it is essential that you can provide a clear rationale for the care you give. You need to be able to tell the patient/client/student why an intervention or procedure is required and be able to provide a clear rationale. This is part of evidence-based practice.

But providing a rationale alone is not enough . . .

Being able to provide a clear rationale for the care you give is essential but not quite sufficient.

 An EBP approach requires that we ensure our rationale is not only clear *but also* up to date and based on the best available evidence.

In other words, you need to be able to defend your practice and ensure that you have a good rationale for the actions you have taken. Wherever possible, your rationale should be based on the **best possible evidence**, although what we mean by 'evidence' is very broadly defined and will be different in varying circumstances. There are **lots of different types of evidence** that we can draw on to underpin practice and we will discuss these throughout this book. Often the best evidence will be research studies or, better still, a review of all research studies undertaken in an area, often referred to as a review or systematic review. Look again at the example above about the social work student on placement and the advice given to the family with the child who had behavioural problems. The multidisciplinary team knew about the provision of groups that might help the parents cope with the behaviour of the child. However, this alone is not enough. Where public resources and services are limited, we need to be as sure as possible that a support group is likely to be useful and effective if made available to the parents. We need to make sure that the **evidence** or **rationale** for the care we provide is **robust.** In this case, the social worker explained her rationale to the student. This rationale was based on a large review of many different research studies that had evaluated the impact of parenting groups for children with behavioural difficulties (Barlow 2016). A review of research studies is usually referred to as a literature review or systematic review. The conclusion of this review showed that the vast majority of research had identified that the provision of parenting classes was beneficial to both the subsequent behaviour of the child and the stress and anxiety of the family unit.

Defining evidence-based practice

Evidence-based practice is not just about evidence. David Sackett, founder of the NHS Research and Development Centre for Evidence-Based Medicine in Oxford, and his colleagues defined evidence-based practice as follows:

Evidence-based practice is: 'The conscientious and judicious use of current best evidence in conjunction with clinical expertise and patient values to guide health [and social] care decisions'. (Sackett et al. 2000: 71–72)

There are many definitions of evidence-based practice. Yet the definitions are all broadly similar. Sackett and colleagues emphasized the strong link between evidence-based practice and the decisions we make in our everyday practice. Decisions should be clearly stated and well thought through (judicious), and use evidence sensibly and carefully. They also emphasize the role of **professional judgement** and **patient/ client preference** – the other components of evidence-based practice that will be explored further later in this chapter.

Evidence alone is not enough – it should be supplemented with the judgement of the practitioner and the wishes of the patient or client. This was echoed by Dawes et al., in the Sicily Statement, in which the role of both tacit and explicit knowledge of healthcare professionals is emphasized in addition to the views of the patient or client:

> *Evidence Based Practice (EBP) requires that decisions about health and social care are based on the best available, current, valid and relevant evidence. These decisions should be made by those receiving care, informed by the tacit and explicit knowledge of those providing care, within the context of available resources.*
>
> (Dawes et al. 2005: 7)

A recent definition by Melnyk and Fineout-Overholt (2014: 3) emphasizes the link between evidence-based practice and problem solving. They state that evidence-based practice is

> *... [a] lifelong problem-solving approach to clinical practice that integrates:*
>
> * *A systematic search for as well as critical appraisal and synthesis of the most relevant and best research (i.e. external evidence) to answer a burning clinical question.*
> * *One's own clinical expertise which includes internal evidence generated from outcomes management or quality improvement projects, a thorough patient assessment, and evaluation and use of available resources necessary to achieve patient outcomes.*
> * *Patient preferences and values.*

In order to emphasize the role of professional judgement and patient or client preference within evidence-based practice, other terms have emerged. Nevo and Slomin-Nevo adopt the term **evidence-informed practice** (EIP) and emphasize that the principles of evidence and professional judgement should be central to our approach to patient or client care. Thus they argue that evidence-informed practice should be understood as:

> *... excluding non-scientific prejudices and superstitions, but also as leaving ample room for clinical experience as well as the constructive and imaginative judgements of practitioners and clients who are in constant interaction and dialogue with one another.*
>
> (Nevo and Slomin-Nevo 2011: 1)

Many commentators, such as Woodbury and Kuhnke (2014) and Miles and Loughlin (2011) argue for the need for a person-centred approach to care delivery. Miles and Loughlin (2011: 534) emphasize that personalized models of care should be *informed by* but not *based on* evidence. A person-centred approach to care delivery is also the basis of the concept of 'values-based practice'. Fulford et al. (2012) describe how evidence-based treatment possibilities should be in tune with the values of the particular patient or client in the prevailing circumstances. They further describe values-based practice incorporating four clinical skills: awareness, reasoning, knowledge, and communication (p. 206).

Where do you think the balance should lie between the health and social care provider making a decision and that decision being made by those in receipt of care?

Different terminology used

We have defined evidence-based practice as we understand it. However, there are many different terms that refer to the broader concept of 'evidence-based practice' or 'evidence-informed practice'. Among others, these include:

- Evidence-based medicine
- Research-based practice
- Evidence-based nursing
- Evidence-based physiotherapy
- Evidence-based dietetics
- Evidence-based midwifery
- Evidence-based occupational therapy.

If you were to study the exact components of each of these, you might find slight variations in emphasis in the definitions but you would find general agreement that all definitions include **use of evidence** combined with **professional opinion and patient or client preference**. We would argue that despite differences in nuance, these terms share the same overriding philosophy.

Exploring the components of evidence-based practice

There are three main components of evidence-based practice:
- *Use of evidence.*
- *Clinical or professional judgement.*
- *Patient/client preference.*

Let us now look at each of these ideas in turn.

Use of evidence

We have shown in the examples above how practitioners have used evidence to justify the rationale for the care they provide and how evidence is a central component of evidence-based practice. We need evidence and we should seek the best available evidence. In Chapter 6, we discuss how you can tell if the evidence is strong or not. What has changed in recent years is the acknowledgement that the term 'evidence' is quite broad and you could be looking at many diverse sources of evidence and other information to justify your practice. We will discuss the type of evidence you might come across in detail in Chapter 4 but in summary, the term 'evidence' does not simply refer to research done in a laboratory under strict controlled conditions! Different types of research provide evidence depending on the situation, although the best evidence for our professional practice is usually some type of research evidence – if it is available.

 Consider how you would value the findings of a well-conducted piece of research that compared different ways of quitting smoking to an anecdotal account from one person who had tried to quit and had failed to do so.

You can usually recognize a piece of research by where it is published and the way it is presented. Research is usually written up in a paper published in one of the professional journals. Professional journals, such as *Addiction, Journal of Advanced Nursing,* and *Journal of Social, Behavioral, and Health Sciences* are often considered to be the gold standard of professional information because the material has always been **peer-reviewed** and checked before acceptance for publication. A research study usually starts with a question – called the **research question** – or clear **aims** or a **hypothesis,** which the researchers then seek to answer or investigate using a **method** that is clearly stated in the research paper, followed by the **results or findings** and then a **discussion** of what these results are likely to mean.

Ideally, we would not rely on a single research study, but a review of studies (sometimes called a literature review or a **systematic review**). A review of evidence provides stronger evidence than a single study because identifying the whole range of studies about a topic will be more reliable than the results of just one, which might be misleading or provide an inaccurate picture.

The study referred to earlier by Barlow (2016) is an example of a systematic review. The term 'systematic' refers to a review of the literature or evidence that has been carried out in a systematic and rigorous way and such reviews generally provide high-quality evidence. The most widely known systematic reviews are those produced by the **Cochrane** and **Campbell Collaborations**, which we refer to later in this book.

If you come across a review published by either the Cochrane or Campbell Collaboration, then you have probably located evidence of good quality.

If there are no systematic reviews or literature reviews on the topic you are interested in, then the next best thing is to find a research study or several studies on your topic. *The types of study you are looking for will depend on the focus or question you wish to address*; the different types of research will be discussed in Chapter 4. There are many different approaches to research and we will consider these later. It is important to emphasize that different types of research are required depending on what you want to find out (i.e. your question). It is not helpful to say that one type of research is 'better' than another. However, it is possible and necessary to make a judgement about the quality of the research and whether it has been carried out well or not; we will discuss how to do this in Chapter 6.

It is sometimes the case that there is **insufficient research evidence** upon which to base practice or the research evidence you come across is **inconclusive** or of **poor quality**. There might be a lack of evidence because it would be unethical to undertake research in the particular area you are interested in. It may also be the case that there is research but it **does not directly apply** to your particular area or your particular patient or client situation, and you need to use your **professional judgement** as to whether the research can be applied in the context in which you are working. There will also be times when you need to draw on alternative sources of evidence other than research evidence alone.

However, it is important to note that it is **research** that often – but not always – provides the strongest **evidence** upon which we base our practice and is at the heart of evidence-based practice. However, research evidence alone is not enough for your practice. This is why the definitions of evidence-based practice include reference to your clinical/professional judgement and patient or client preference. We will now address the former component of evidence-based practice.

Clinical/professional judgement and intuition

Our own professional or clinical judgement is vital for providing an evidence-based approach to care. In their early discussion of evidence-based practice, Sackett and colleagues (1996) describe how evidence can inform decisions about practice, but cannot replace professional expertise and judgement. They argue that this clinical/professional expertise is used to determine whether the available evidence should be applied to the individual patient/client at all and, if so, if it should be used to inform our decision-making. Professional or clinical judgement includes 'the assessment of alternatives' (Thompson et al. 2013: 1721). Thompson et al. (2013) emphasize the importance of considering alternative courses of action and recognize the potential for harm when an inappropriate assessment is made. It is important that all the evidence we use is professionally evaluated, because every patient or client context is unique and all clinical situations are, to some degree, uncertain.

Standing (2014) describes how clinical judgement is informed by a range of evidence, from patient observation to published research studies. In emergencies, there may be a greater need for clinical or professional judgement, as there will be no time to gather the best available evidence and our judgement will focus on how we can meet the immediate needs of the patient or client in front of us. When it is possible to plan care more thoroughly in advance, this should involve the writing of guidelines or protocols for emergency situations, and so the best available evidence will be used to inform care even in clinical and professional situations that require prompt decision-making.

Professional or clinical judgement may also be used alongside intuition. Intuition is often referred to as gut feeling – 'just knowing'.

- There appears to be a close relationship between experience and intuition.
- Intuition is grounded in both knowledge and experience in making judgements.

(Benner 1984; Benner and Tanner 1987)

Standing (2014) argues that intuition can be useful when needing to make a clinical judgement in emergencies. Indeed, Benner and Tanner argued this back in 1987 when they described how intuitive knowledge and analytical reasoning are not opposed to each other – they can and do work together.

Clinical/professional judgement is also important if there is insufficient evidence, or the evidence does not refer to the specific patient/client you are looking after. Thus, a judgement needs to be made as to how relevant the evidence we have is to the particular **context**, **complexity**, and **individuality** of the patient or client.

Where there is no reliable research evidence, the judgement of the prac-
titioner may form the best evidence.

What evidence is there to support using intuition?

The importance of professional judgement and intuition was reinforced by a literature review (McGraughey et al. 2009) that gathered together the evidence about the use of checklists versus professional judgement/ intuition in the nursing assessment of patients whose condition had rapidly deteriorated. The use of checklists to trigger nursing staff to refer a patient for urgent medical attention has become widely used. They are promoted as a way of standardizing the referral for urgent medical attention and, in theory at least, replace nurses' intuition with a more objective approach. This is in addition to an assessment of the patient's vital signs, which is a check on whether or not the patient's condition has deteriorated. Whether the use of these checklists has made hospitals a safer place for patients whose condition deteriorates has been widely researched. Thus, McGraughey and colleagues (2009) carried out a systematic review to compare the results of all of these studies. In their review, they found that nurses' intuition was as reliable a trigger for seeking medical help as the use of a checklist or tool. Douw et al. (2015) reported similar findings in their systematic review exploring nurses' use of intuition versus measurement of vital signs in recognizing deterioration in patients. This might be why some health and social care practitioners state that their **professional work is an art as well as a science**, and it incorporates a human element that cannot be reduced to just the application of research knowledge to patient/ client care. This can be described as clinical or professional judgement.

It is important to emphasize that intuition and experience are used in con-junction with an evidence-based approach. Intuition and/or pattern matching are useful aids to good clinical reasoning but only when used as prompts to engage in analytical reasoning (Ruth-Sahd 2014).

Using evidence without professional judgement can lead to formulaic
care, while using professional judgement without available evidence can lead to the perpetuation of outdated practice. The two should work together!

So far, we have argued that evidence-based practice requires more than 'raw' evidence. It requires clinical or professional judgement. This may be based on intuition and/or experience so that the evidence can be applied appropriately in practice. Now let's look at patient/client preferences and what role they play in evidence-based practice.

Patient/client preference

There is also a third component – that the patient's/client's preference must be acknowledged and their informed **consent** sought before commencing any intervention. If all the best evidence and clinical or professional judgement pointed towards an intervention or therapy that the patient/client did not accept, then it ought not be carried out. This concept is well established in English law (*R v Blau* 1975).

Discover what your professional body says about consent before undertaking care or an intervention.

In addition, there has been a debate recently about the importance of shared decision-making and increased patient/client involvement in the health and social care context. This is discussed further in Chapter 3.

In legal terms, any care that is delivered without the patient's/client's consent may be unlawful. Children under 16 cannot give their consent unless they are considered competent under the Fraser Guidelines (Griffiths 2017). If the patient is temporarily (in an emergency) or permanently unable to consent, care for the patient/client should be delivered that is in their best interests.

Care for those who are unable to consent is determined in the Mental Capacity Act (Department of Constitutional Affairs 2005, implemented 2007) [see http://www.legislation.gov.uk/ukpga/2005/9/contents].

The Mental Capacity Act:

- Presumes capacity
- Reinforces the right of individuals to be supported to make decisions
- Reinforces the right of individuals to make eccentric or unwise decisions
- Reinforces that anything done for or on behalf of people without capacity must be done 'in their best interests'
- Reinforces that anything done for or on behalf of people without capacity should be least restrictive of rights and freedoms.

Check you are fully aware of the principles regarding informed consent.

There is some evidence to suggest that urgent care is sometimes delayed because practitioners are not aware that they can deliver care that is in the best interests of a patient or client who cannot consent (Variend 2012).

Some patient/clients really want to be involved in any decisions relating to their care. Others trust the practitioner to make the best possible decision on their behalf. This is a big responsibility and we need to be well informed as to what might be the best option for our patient/client. There are many decision aids available to help patients who need to make treatment choices.

The main point to remember is that patient preference must be considered when providing evidence-based care. While patients cannot demand care that is not available, equally care cannot be delivered without their consent and to do so would be to risk professional misconduct and be in breach of the law unless the patient or client lacks the ability to consent.

Duty of candour

With regards to patient/client involvement and adopting an open and honest approach, the Care Quality Commission's (2016) Regulation 20 discusses 'Duty of Candour' and asserts that care providers should ensure openness and transparency with service users and their advocates. The Commission has identified specific requirements that must be followed when things go wrong with care and treatment, including providing truthful information, support, and apologizing when things go wrong.

> For nurses and midwives, there is additional guidance on the Professional Duty of Candour (NMC 2015a) produced by the Nursing and Midwifery Council in collaboration with the General Medical Council. Specifically, section 76:d states with regard to joint decision-making that any evidence of previously expressed patient/client preferences should be considered [see https://www.nmc.org.uk/standards/guidance/the-professional-duty-of-candour/].
>
> The guidance should be read alongside the Code (NMC 2015b).

Part of this is to ensure that both the risks and benefits of treatment or care are explained to the patient or client, which links very well with the notion of using evidence-based practice, particularly when we consider patient/client consent, their involvement, and preferences.

Consequences of not taking an evidence-based approach

Although delivery of the **best possible care** is the main driver behind evidence-based practice, there are consequences for you as a practitioner if you are not able to explain your care decisions and these will now be discussed.

Example from practice

Imagine you are the parent of a baby who has been invited for the MMR vaccination. You discuss the media scare surrounding this vaccination with the nurse practitioner. The nurse is not familiar with the limitations of the original paper or with the vast body of medical evidence that has subsequently found the vaccination to be safe. She remains cautious about the use of the vaccination and hence does not reassure you that the vaccination is safe. You decline the vaccination and your baby remains at risk from measles, mumps, and rubella. Yet the advice given was not evidence-based.

Accountability

In the example above, you would feel justified about considering a complaint against the practitioner who was not up to date or confident discussing current evidence. If you did make a complaint, the practitioner would then have to justify why this information was given. This would be very difficult to do, if not impossible.

 As a health or social care practitioner, you are accountable to your manager or university (if you are a student), your professional organization, and to the law.

This means that you must be able to justify and give a clear account of and rationale for your practice. Failure to do this can result in professional misconduct.

- Students are accountable to their higher education institution and when in practice ought to be supervised directly or indirectly by a registered practitioner.

- Registered practitioners are accountable to their professional body and their employers.
- We are all accountable to the law.

You can see that when you are called to account for your practice, you will only be able to do so if you have administered care that is based on the best available evidence. You will not be able to account for care that is based on old or weak evidence.

Find out what your professional body, college *or* association *says about your accountability and evidence-based practice.*

In the United Kingdom, these are as follows:

For **allied health professions and social workers**, including occupational therapists, physiotherapists, operating department practitioners, dieticians, paramedics, radiographers, speech and language therapists, art therapists, chiropodists/podiatrists, clinical scientists, orthoptists, prosthetists, and orthotists: the **Health and Care Professions Council** (HCPC). The HCPC publishes *Standards of Conduct, Performance and Ethics* [available at: http://www.hpc-uk.org/aboutregistration/standards/]. They state that 'You must keep your knowledge and skills up to date and relevant to your scope of practice through continuing professional development' (HCPC 2016: 7).

For nurses and midwives: the **Nursing and Midwifery Council (NMC)**. The NMC publishes *The Code: Professional standards of practice and behaviour for nurses and midwives* [available at: https://www.nmc.org. uk/standards/code/]. The Code (NMC 2015b: 7) requires all practitioners to 'practise in line with the best available evidence'. In addition, nurses should:

> ... *make sure that any information or advice given is evidence-based, including information relating to using any healthcare products or services, and maintain the knowledge and skills you need for safe and effective practice.*
>
> (NMC 2015b: 7)

Therefore, if you are called upon to account for your practice, you must be able to provide a sound rationale for why you acted as you did. If you are only able to say 'I was told to do this' or 'I've always done it this way', your practice will look very poor indeed! Students are expected to work towards these standards in order to obtain registration and failure to do so may affect progression towards qualification.

Individual colleges and associations often produce professional guidance and you should access their websites to see what relates to your own profession.

 Do you think the practitioner referred to earlier would be found guilty of professional misconduct owing to the mis-information she gave regarding childhood vaccinations?

Clinical governance

In addition to accountability via the professional governing bodies in the UK, health and social care practitioners are also accountable to the organization in which they work through the concept of clinical governance. On clinical governance, the Department of Health [http://www.dh.gov.uk/health/2011/09/clinical-governance/] states:

> ***Clinical governance*** describes the structures, processes and culture needed to ensure that healthcare organisations – and all individuals within them – can assure the quality of the care they provide and are continuously seeking to improve it.
>
> (Department of Health 2011)

The mechanisms of clinical governance are recognized by many health and social care organizations internationally but may be referred to by different terminology. Governance provides a framework through which organizations are accountable for improving the quality of services and maintaining high standards (Gottwald and Lansdown 2014). In the UK, this was particularly apparent when the Mid Staffordshire NHS Foundation Trust public enquiry (Francis 2013) highlighted systematic failure to provide adequate care and the importance of governance and accountability.

Campaigns on improving safety have helped practitioners to provide safe care. For example, 'Sign up to Safety' (NHS England 2014) is a national initiative to help NHS organizations and their staff achieve their patient safety aspirations and care for their patients in the safest way possible. There are five Sign up to Safety pledges and more detail can be found on the NHS England website [https://www.england.nhs.uk/signuptosafety/about/].

The purpose of clinical governance is to ensure that the institution – in addition to the individual practitioner – is accountable for the care that its service provides.

In addition, the **Essence of Care** benchmarking statements have been designed to contribute to the introduction of clinical governance at local level. The benchmarking process outlined in 'The essence of care' statements, 'helps practitioners to take a structured approach to sharing and comparing practice, enabling them to identify the **best practice** and to develop action plans to remedy poor practice' (Department of Health 2010). [These documents are available at https://www.gov.uk/government/publications/essence-of-care-2010, while the Appendix to this book provides more specific information.]

Non-NHS organizations also have standards and quality assurance initiatives.

Legal considerations

Finally, in addition to accountability to the relevant professional body and employing institution, as a registered practitioner you are accountable to the law. The main area of law in the UK that is likely to be of relevance to those working within health and social care is the tort of negligence. Being able to justify the care that you give may protect you or your organization from a claim in negligence. There is a developing culture of litigation and claims against health and social care organizations. Patients or clients who are unhappy about the care they receive can make a claim in negligence if they have suffered harm as a result of that care. The National Health Service Litigation Authority (NHSLA) handles negligence claims and works to improve risk management practices in the NHS [see http://www.nhsla.com/Pages/Home.aspx]. Clinical governance, discussed earlier, includes several measures to ensure we provide safe and effective care.

Let's return to the example above of the nurse providing mis-information about the MMR vaccination. Say that the worst does happen and your child contracts measles from which he has lasting complications. To make a successful claim in negligence against a health and social care provider, the patient/client has to demonstrate that the healthcare provider failed in their duty to provide care and that this failure led to harm. The courts have consistently ruled that such a failure occurs if the health or social care provider has provided care that is not evidence-based. In this case, failure to provide up-to-date information about the safety of a vaccination programme is likely to amount to a breach of duty and might lead to a claim of negligence. Under the current system, you can only make a claim in negligence if you have suffered harm.

 Being able to provide a good rationale or explanation for your practice is an essential component of the concept of 'evidence-based practice' and could even prevent you from becoming involved in any legal proceedings.

Therefore, you can see that you are less likely to make errors or give the wrong information to your service users if you follow recommendations for best practice and have a sound rationale for what you do.

What does evidence-based practice mean to me?

So far in this chapter, we have introduced the concept of evidence-based practice and why we believe it to be so important. We have used examples from professional health and social care practice to illustrate this and the likely implications that can arise from following a 'non-evidence-based' approach.

Throughout this book, we will look in more detail at how you might adopt an evidence-based approach. The following provides an illustration of how an evidence-based approach may be used in professional practice and we identify where in this book we discuss the **five stages of using an evidence-based approach**.

1 **Identify what you need to find out:** this may be information or evidence about the best care for an individual patient or client or more generally for public health.
2 **Search for the most appropriate evidence:** this is usually research evidence but could be another form of evidence, as we will discuss in Chapter 5.
3 **Try to work out if the evidence you find is any good:** we refer to this process as 'critical appraisal of the evidence' and we will discuss how we assess the quality of evidence in Chapter 6.
4 **Incorporate the evidence into a strategy for action:** if the evidence is good enough, refer to your professional judgement and patient or client preference. We will discuss this further in Chapter 7.
5 **Evaluate the effects of any decisions and action taken:** this will be discussed further in Chapter 7.

Examples from practice

Example 1: You notice that several practitioners carry out an intervention differently. You wonder why this is and when you ask questions in your professional practice, you get different answers!

Example 2: Alternatively, say you have been asked to write an essay or discuss a case study on a given scenario discussing what you did and why you did it.

For both of these examples, you would need to take an evidence-based approach and ask yourself: **'What is the evidence for the way the care was undertaken?'**

To answer this question, you would first need to **search for** and **locate** the appropriate evidence. You might find a wide range of different research studies, case studies, guidelines, literature reviews or opinion articles. You would then need to **judge the quality** of the evidence you find and whether it is relevant to your problem or issue. You would probably consider any research that you find to be of more value than someone's personal view. This evidence should then be **applied** to the care of the patient or client, whose needs initiated the question, taking into account their preference and your clinical or professional judgement. The **resources** available may also need to be considered at this point. You may then want to **evaluate** the effectiveness of your intervention in the circumstances with that particular patient or client.

We will cover how to ask the right question, how to search for the evidence, and how to judge the value and quality of different types of evidence in more detail later in this book.

This is evidence-based practice in practice!

It is important to find the right evidence to underpin your practice and this book will show you how best to do that. You can see that carrying out an intervention or approach because it has 'always been done' or acting because something is expected of you is not enough. You need to ensure that there are strong reasons and evidence rather than acting out of a sense of amend tradition or ritual. This is not to say that traditional practices are necessarily outdated or to be avoided at all costs. Nor is experience alone to be disregarded. It is just that nowadays, as practitioners, we have a wealth of research available to us that can inform how we should proceed in practice, while considering professional judgement and patient or client preference. Given that we have this opportunity, we need to ensure that we use it for the best outcomes for our patients and clients.

In summary

In this chapter, we have discussed the meaning of the term evidence-based practice. We hope that you now think there is a logical argument for health and social care to be evidence-based. After all, who would want to receive outdated care from a practitioner who could not account for it, rather than care that is based on the best available evidence combined with professional judgement and patient/client involvement?

In the remainder of this book, we will consider why practice needs evidence and what we mean by evidence. We will then consider different research approaches that you might encounter. We will discuss how to search for evidence and then consider how to determine whether it is any good or not. We will then consider the thorny question of implementing evidence-based practice. Before that, however, we will consider in more detail why evidence-based practice has become so important to our practice today.

Key points

1 There are several reasons why we need to adopt EBP:
  (a) to ensure best practice
  (b) for our professional accountability
  (c) to avoid litigation/negligence claims.
2 Evidence-based practice incorporates using the best available evidence, clinical or professional judgement, and patient/client preference in our decision-making.
3 Evidence-based practice should not replace intuition or experience in our practice but should be used alongside them.

Quiz questions

1 What are the three main components of evidence-based practice?
2 How might you consider involving your patient/client preferences when making decisions?
3 What does your own professional body/organization say about your accountability to deliver evidence-based practice?

2 Evidence-based practice and the information and communication revolution

- *Moving away from ritual and traditional approaches*
- *The developing research culture worldwide*
- *The on-going information and communications revolution*
- *Why is there so much information available?*
- *So how does this 'information revolution' affect me?*
- *In summary*
- *Key points*
- *Quiz questions*

In this chapter, we will:

- Explore the development of evidence-based practice
- Explore the on-going information revolution
- Discuss how this has assisted the transition from reliance on tradition and ritual in our practice towards the use of evidence.

So far, we have argued that evidence-based practice is an essential approach to the delivery of health and social care. We have discussed how evidence-based practice is practice based upon a sound, up-to-date rationale and your own clinical or professional judgement and that it takes into account the patient's/client's wishes. We have also argued that although there are many definitions of evidence-based practice and different terms to describe the concept, the central message is consistent throughout:

> **Use of evidence combined with professional judgement and patient preference should result in high-quality care.**

We have also discussed how as a student or registered practitioner you need to be able to give reasons for the care you deliver. These ideas might seem totally sensible and logical to you as you read this book. However, it is important to acknowledge that although evidence-based practice has been around since the 1990s (Greenhalgh 2014), it has not always been accepted as the norm and there are still some practitioners who are yet to embrace the concept, due to lack of understanding, motivation or skill.

Moving away from ritual and tradition towards an evidence-based approach

For many hundreds of years, health and social care practices were based on experience, trial and error, tradition and ritual. Even where an interest in science and research existed, communication was limited so that it was difficult to circulate new ideas and developments, especially on a large scale.

 For many centuries, the concepts of experience, tradition, *and* ritual *dominated health and social care.*

Practitioners in the past largely relied on trial and error, following doctor's orders, protocols, experience, ritual, and what was accepted practice. A culture of research and development had yet to be firmly established within health and social care contexts. You are probably familiar with some of the more popular rituals that were practised. Within health and social care, there is today considerable international movement of staff and so 'traditional ways of working' may stem from both national and international custom and practice.

 Think back to practices that you have previously carried out that are now considered unhelpful or even harmful. If you are a student or new to your profession, ask your practice assessor/mentor if they know of any.

Let's take some examples of practices that have been adhered to that do not have an evidence base to support them.

Examples from practice

Example 1: Smith and Judge (2016) discuss how the technique of pericardial thump was taught as part of standard cardio-pulmonary resuscitation (CPR) training for many years. This procedure was based on anecdotal reports and could result in sternal fracture, osteomyelitis, stroke, and rhythm deterioration.

Example 2: For many years, Cumming and Henry's (1961) 'theory of disengagement' influenced social care practice by promoting care based in institutions and ultimately encouraging inactivity of the elderly who lived in them. The lack of evidence behind this theory has gradually been exposed and older members of society are now encouraged to continue to be active and engaged citizens. In the light of more recent evidence, there has been a Twitter campaign called #EndPjParalysis with the aim of getting patients out of their pyjamas and moving! (Mckew 2017).

From these two examples, it is clear that the absence of an appropriate evidence base led to practices that were harmful. This is not to say there was a complete absence of research but where research did exist, it is widely acknowledged that it took a very long time for it to be adopted in practice. To take another example, one of the early studies on the treatment of scurvy, undertaken by surgeon James Lind in 1753 with members of the Royal Navy, identified that citrus fruit could reduce the incidence of scurvy. Records suggest it took another forty years before the Navy routinely gave citrus fruits to its sailors and a further sixty years before the use of citrus fruit was encouraged in the general population (Dunn 1997).

Gradually, as a culture of research developed within health and social care, more practices were founded on research and became 'evidence-based'. The following example illustrates how the development of an evidence-based approach can lead to the reduction of interventions that may be unpleasant or harmful, and for which there is no solid evidence base.

Example from practice

Greenway (2014) discusses how the incorrect administration of intramuscular injections fits into the description of ritualistic practice.

She notes that if educators and mentors do not keep up to date and change practice despite the publication of evidence-based guidelines and resources, then ritualistic practices will continue.

Can you identify an area of your own profession where a change in practice has been recommended based on changes in evidence?

The developing research culture worldwide

The research culture within health and social care has become stronger over the past few decades. The concept of 'research-based practice' evolved and practitioners increasingly began to search for a research base for the care they delivered that previously might have been given according to tradition, experience, and following orders without question. At the same time, **research education** became a main component of university courses for health and social care professionals both at undergraduate and postgraduate level. Demand for research to underpin practice has increased as more professions have moved their registered professional roles towards **higher education** rather than on-the-job training or apprenticeship.

Over time, the term 'research-based practice' has been replaced by 'evidence-based practice' in order to incorporate the influence of professional judgement and patient preference, as discussed in Chapter 1. Now we see the influence of evidence-based practice on a worldwide scale, as recognition of the value of research and evidence impacts on health systems and public health internationally.

For example, the Cochrane Collaboration and its sister organization the Campbell Collaboration are both widely acknowledged to be world leaders in producing high-quality, credible information to inform decision-making within health and social care. Since 2011, the Cochrane Collaboration has been an official partner of the **World Health Organization** (WHO). This partnership ensures that there is an integration of research evidence and policy. This collaboration between sectors and the high-quality research between the two organizations contributes to producing the necessary evidence to ensure policies in all sectors contribute to improving health and health equity [see http://www.cochrane.org/about-us/our-partners-and-funders/world-health-organization].

The Cochrane Collaboration also has a link with **Wikipedia** that was formalized in 2014. Members of the Cochrane Collaboration actively engage with Wikipedia in order to enhance the evidence base of the information provided. On their webpage [http://www.cochrane.org/about-us/our-partners-and-funders/wikipedia], Cochrane note that there are more than 180 million views per month of articles relating to health, of which less than 1 per cent had been peer-reviewed. Cochrane considers it has a role in working towards transforming the quality and content of health evidence available online and the inclusion of relevant evidence within all Wikipedia medical articles.

The result of the growth of these and other sources is that we now have a large evidence pool upon which to base our practice, although some areas of health and social care are very well researched while others remain under-researched.

There is a YouTube video you can view showing the challenges faced around the world in relation to the Cochrane 'Strategy to 2020' [see https://youtu.be/uaHZLrVGpE0].

On the partnership between Cochrane and Wikipedia (discussed above), see the discussion online about opening up medical information to a wider audience in many different languages [see https://www.youtube.com/watch?v=tUrwbu8At7Q].

The Cochrane (2016) 'Strategy to 2020' aims to put Cochrane evidence at the heart of health decision-making all over the world. It is based on achieving four key goals:

- Goal 1: To produce relevant, current high-quality evidence from systematic reviews and evidence synthesis
- Goal 2: To ensure that the evidence produced is relevant and accessible worldwide
- Goal 3: To promote Cochrane as a leading source of evidence to inform healthcare decisions
- Goal 4: To develop and sustain an international Cochrane Organization to be effective, accountable, inclusive, diverse, and transparent. It will use guiding principles and the motivation and talent of its contributors.

In addition to the global approaches identified above, below are some specific examples of evidence that have contributed to an evidence-based approach and changes in practice.

Examples of evidence contributing to an evidence-based approach

Example 1: Birnbaum and Saini (2012) undertook a review of qualitative studies exploring whether children wished to be involved in custody decisions post separation or divorce and found that children generally want to be engaged in the decision-making process regarding custody and access, even if they are not making the final decisions. The suggestion is that social workers ought to listen to the views of children in this aspect of their work.

Example 2: In a large randomized controlled trial, Aveyard et al. (2016) looked at the effectiveness of different health promotion activities within primary care aimed at patients who were overweight. They found that when the GP brought up the topic of weight loss with a patient and subsequently invited him or her to attend a commercial weight-loss programme, the patient lost significantly more weight than the controls with whom the GP had a general discussion about weight management. As a result, GPs now have a strategy with a clear evidence base for helping those with weight management problems.

Example 3: The third example comes from the medical treatment of breast cancer but is used here because it illustrates the points we are making. If we look back fifty years, the best-known treatment for breast cancer was a full mastectomy, which entailed the total removal of the breast. This was the standard treatment for many years. In the 1970s, scientists began to consider whether such radical treatment was indeed the best option and commenced trials to compare whether removal of the malignant lump would be as effective as removal of the whole breast. Many very large studies (known as randomized controlled trials, which we discuss in Chapter 5) were conducted across Europe and the USA and the results of these studies confirmed that it was both safe and effective to remove just the lump rather than the whole breast (Fisher et al. 2002). As a result of these many studies, practitioners were able to inform patient/clients that a full mastectomy was no longer necessary and the best possible treatment, in most instances, was removal of the lump only. Thus, as a result of these studies, it was possible to establish best practice for the management of breast cancer. The results of these studies led to radical changes in the way that breast cancer was managed.

These are just some examples of research that has led to changes in practice and has contributed to the development of evidence-based practice.

The on-going information revolution

The amount and range of information available to practitioners are now so vast that it seems impossible to keep on top of. This information is also expanding on a daily basis.

As a health or social care practitioner, you may feel overwhelmed by the amount of information, of varying quality, which relates to many different specialties and topics. As vast amounts of research and other information become more readily available, it is increasingly hard to keep abreast of new developments. Indeed, one group of researchers calculated the number of new journal articles published in a particular area on a weekly basis and came to the conclusion that keeping up to date, let alone being an 'expert' on a topic, had become an impossible expectation (Fraser and Dunstan 2010).

Think how much easier it must have been before so much evidence was available upon which to base health and social care practice. Maybe there were one or two textbooks to read, rather than the many Internet sources, journals, videos, and e-books that are available today.

Why is so much information available?

There are two main reasons why there is so much available evidence:

- *Increased demand for research and more/better quality research being produced*
- *Information is more widely available from the Internet and other sources.*

Increased demand for research and more and better quality research is being produced

We have discussed the increasing demand for research and the development of the concept of evidence-based practice, which has arisen as health and social care practitioners move away from a traditional approach to care delivery towards an evidence-based approach. This has led to an enormous number of publications and the development of research organizations such as the **Cochrane Collaboration** and **Campbell Collaboration** as mentioned earlier in this chapter and in Chapter 1. You only have to look at the titles of journals in any library collection to see the range of journals that relate to a particular professional field. In addition, some of these journals may be published on a weekly or monthly basis. It can seem an impossible task to keep up to date with new developments, even within your own area, without developing strategies for managing the information that we will discuss later in this chapter.

However, this is not to say that you will always find evidence to underpin your practice. There are important areas that have not been researched. All research needs to be approved by appropriate ethical bodies, and it can take years after the successful award of a research grant before any research is undertaken. This is because research is a complex and lengthy process that can take some time to get started.

Examples from practice

Example 1: A recent NHS briefing paper [available at http://www.hra.nhs.uk/documents/2016/02point-care-trials-meeting-3-dec-15-background-paper.pdf] describes the lack of evidence for many therapies for children, as clinical trials are undertaken on the adult population. Treatments tested on adults have been adapted for use with children without being investigated specifically among this client group.

Example 2: In a letter to the *British Medical Journal*, Heneghan et al. (2016) discuss the lack of evidence for fertility investigations and emphasize the possible role of the National Institute for Health and Care Excellence (NICE), which could identify gaps and advise how these could be addressed.

Information is more widely available on the Internet, mobile devices, and social media

The second reason for the escalation in available information is the dramatic rise in **information technology**, leading to the widespread availability and increased accessibility of information, and improved ways of sharing information, such as via social media. Before the advent of this technology, libraries contained hard-bound indexes and volumes of the journals that were likely to be most relevant to their students. Practitioners would probably subscribe locally to relevant professional journals and even have their own departmental libraries. This restricted the range of what was available. Consequently, there were always a large number of journals that were not available to staff and students or available only through inter-library loan. This made it difficult and expensive to access relevant information.

With the advent of online libraries, databases, and journals, students and practitioners now have access to many thousands of journals and e-books in addition to websites and other sources of information and references. The way both professionals and the public communicate and access information is changing rapidly from a planned, static approach to the expectation that information can be accessed spontaneously, anywhere and immediately using mobile devices.

Use of social media as a source of evidence

In addition to the increase in available information, there have also been changes to the way it can be accessed. Traditional methods of information delivery have been supplemented by the use of **social media**. This has been widely embraced as a positive culture within health and social care, opening up new ways of communication and generating ideas (Sinclair et al. 2015) and even assessment (Jones et al. 2016). In an integrative review, Rolls et al. (2016) explored how healthcare professionals use social media to create virtual communities, and found that there is emerging evidence that professionals share knowledge using social media. However, it should be noted that the evidence suggests that clinicians prefer to use social media that allows them to communicate within their own profession or discipline and within a clinical specialty.

Concern has been expressed that social media can serve as a filter to the information that we access. Viner (2016) and Wong et al. (2016) argue that, paradoxically, instead of increasing our connections and exposure to new ideas, social media can instead lead to a restricted feed of information from sources to which an individual feels an affiliation. Further research is required to evaluate the effects of social media on knowledge distribution in clinical practice and importantly whether patient outcomes are significantly improved. It is thus more important than ever to seek the best available evidence.

Elsewhere (Aveyard et al. 2015), we distinguish between 'easily available evidence' and 'best available evidence', in order to emphasize that the two concepts are very different. With so much information available on the Internet and social media, it can be daunting for students and qualified staff to identify what is the best available evidence, as discussed earlier in this chapter. In Chapter 5, we discuss ways in which we can search for evidence in order to ensure that the best available evidence is located and identified rather than that which most easily comes to hand.

> **Digital media sources** and **social media** play an important role in where and how we get information. In addition, researchers are increasingly considering it as a resource for their research. The National Institute for Health Research (2014) has produced guidance on the use of social media to actively involve people in research [see http://www.invo.org.uk/wp-content/uploads/2014/11/9982-Social-Media-Guide-WEB.pdf].

Learning how to navigate the available information

It is easy to feel overwhelmed by the amount of evidence available on a topic. Information overload has been defined by Kumar and Maskara as the 'difficulty a person can have in comprehending issue [*sic*] and making judgments that are caused by the presence of too much information. Information overload occurs when the amount of input to a system surpasses its processing capacity' (2015: 125).

There are ways to manage information overload, such as using systematic reviews, good quality literature reviews, and research-based guidelines and policy.

Given the increased use of widely available electronic sources, including social media, it is more important than ever to be discerning about the information you use.

One consequence of the information revolution and changes in our culture of communication is that there is a vast amount of unconfirmed and unreliable information out there. A lot of information is misleading, out of date or based on unhelpful assumptions, such as myths, rumours, and 'word on the street'. It is vital that as a practitioner you do not perpetuate these ideas. We discuss how you differentiate good quality evidence from poorer quality evidence in Chapter 6. As a health and social care practitioner, you have to consider all the information and evidence you come across and identify that which is useful to you. Goldacre (2008) illustrates many examples of a non-evidence-based approach in his book entitled *Bad Science*. In this book and on his website [http://www.badscience.net/], Goldacre explores and often exposes health and social care stories that are presented or reported as fact yet are based on very little, inaccurate or no evidence whatsoever.

For example, in his book he dedicates a chapter to homeopathy and, more recently, on his website discusses claims made regarding the role of vitamin supplements in the treatment of HIV and AIDS, and claims that traditional treatments for these diseases are harmful. Goldacre illustrates clearly that the vast amount of information available needs close scrutiny. There is also some concern that practitioners might be tempted to ignore the growing evidence base and continue to use outdated practices.

> Goldacre summarizes some key points in his TED TALK entitled 'Battling Bad Science' [https://www.ted.com/talks/ben_goldacre_battling_bad_science].

Clearly, it is within your role as a health and social care practitioner to get behind the headlines and simple reports so that you are not supporting claims that do not have a sound evidence base.

How does this 'information revolution' affect me?

In short, as practitioners we have a duty to incorporate evidence-based information into our everyday practice to ensure safe and effective patient/client care because we are accountable. In addition to the large amount of information available to us as professionals, our patients/clients are more able to access this information too and so may want to be more involved in decision-making. As the available information increases, it becomes more and more likely that there will be some good quality research available that underpins the care or treatment you deliver. Therefore, if you continue to practise without updating yourself, it is likely that your practice will be out of date. You may then be called to account as to why your practice is out of date or, if you give advice or an intervention that is not based on evidence, you are more likely to be challenged by fellow practitioners, students or patients/clients. With the on-going information revolution, keeping up to date with new ideas and research is arguably more difficult than it was previously.

In summary

The on-going information revolution presents a challenge to all who practise within health and social care. No longer is it acceptable to say '*this is how I've always done this*' and to carry on with an outdated practice in the light of new evidence. The increase in the amount of evidence available and the ways that this can be accessed, together with the demand and drive for research evidence, have led to an expectation and culture in which practice is founded on evidence. As a student or qualified practitioner, you need to be able to justify the care that you give. In the remainder of this book, we will explore how you can best access, evaluate, and make sense of the information that is available to you. In Chapter 5, we discuss how to search for relevant information and evidence. In Chapter 6, we discuss how you can identify whether or not the evidence you access is useful. Finally, in Chapter 7, we discuss strategies for adopting an evidence-based approach, and what the realities of that are like, within the realistic context of busy professional practice.

Key points

1 It is no longer acceptable to base our practice on tradition or ritual.
2 The dramatic rise in the quantity, quality, and availability of information has led to the need to incorporate this information into daily practice.
3 Use of good quality, up-to-date evidence is expected by our patients/ clients and we are accountable for ensuring we use it.

Quiz questions

1   What are the two main reasons for the increase in available information?
2   Identify an area of your own practice that might be based on tradition or ritual and an area of your own practice that has a sound evidence base.
3   How might you personally access high-quality information or evidence in a more manageable way?

3 When do I need to use evidence in my practice?

- *Evidence-based practice and decision-making*
- *The consequences and implications of your decisions*
- *The types of evidence we need when making different decisions*
- *What kinds of evidence are there?*
- *Anecdotal evidence*
- *Research evidence*
- *Research that relates directly to your client or patient group*
- *Research conducted with different client or patient groups or in different settings*
- *What other 'evidence' is out there?*
- *In summary*
- *Key points*
- *Quiz questions*

In this chapter, we will consider:

- When we need to use evidence
- The types of evidence available to help us and our patients/clients make decisions
- What we need to do when there is limited evidence.

So far, we have considered the importance of taking an evidence-based approach and the wealth of information that is available to help you to do that. In this chapter, we consider when you need to use an evidence-based approach. If, before you started reading this book, you thought that evidence-based practice was something that concerned decisions in health and social care at the highest level only, you will now be aware that it is something that affects all practitioners, at all levels of service provision. We discuss what this means in this chapter. We consider how to search for evidence in detail in Chapter 5 and then, in Chapters 6 and 7, discuss in greater detail how you make sense of and apply the evidence you find.

 In simple terms, every time you undertake a professional activity or decision, you need to ask yourself what evidence informs that situation.

Evidence-based practice and decision-making

We make decisions all the time in all professional areas and increasingly we will be supporting our patients/clients in making their own decisions. In 2005, Standing defined decision-making as:

> *A complex process involving information processing, critical thinking, evaluating evidence, applying relevant knowledge, problem solving skills, reflection and clinical judgement to select the best course of action which optimizes a patient/client's health and minimizes any potential harm . . .*
>
> (Standing 2005: 34)

Tiffen et al. (2014: 401) more recently undertook a literature review and used an expert panel to help them define decision-making as:

> *. . . a contextual, continuous, and evolving process, where data are gathered, interpreted, and evaluated in order to select an evidence-based choice of action.*

You can see how these definitions of decision-making require an evidence-based approach – that is, using the best available evidence, together with professional judgement, and taking patient/client preference into consideration. Evaluating the evidence upon which a decision is based is part of professional or clinical judgement, which is a component of evidence-based practice. Standing (2014: 7) makes the link between decision-making and professional judgement when she states that, 'Decision making links judgement to practice by acting on it in choosing from the available options.'

Recognizing that there is more than one possible course of action is part of professional judgement. Hastie and Dawes (2010) state that decision-making consists of three parts:

- There has to be more than one course of action.
- The decision-maker considers the possible or expected outcomes.
- The consequences are assessed of each possible outcome based on personal beliefs and goals.

Tiffin et al. (2014) identify a four-stage, non-linear framework for decision-making that includes:

1 Data gathering
2 Data interpretation
3 Data evaluation and
4 Decision choice.

Data gathering involves getting the best available evidence. This is interpreted and evaluated using professional judgement. The final decision should be made with the patient or client who ought to be involved throughout the whole process. At the centre of their model, Tiffin et al. place the professional, who is able to influence how a situation is appraised or how the complexity of the task is perceived.

Shared decision-making

NHS England (2017) describe **shared decision-making** as:

> . . . a process in which patients, when they reach a decision cross-roads in their health care, can review all the treatment options available to them and participate actively with their healthcare professional in making that decision.

The Health Foundation (2014) discusses how shared decision-making is part of person-centred approaches and includes using evidence-based resources:

> Shared decision making supports patients to make a specific decision such as whether or not to have a diagnostic test, take a course of medication, undertake a mental health recovery programme, or to choose between different types of surgery. It often involves decision support materials – evidence-based information resources, including patient decision aids, brief decision aids, and option grids – that are designed to help individuals weigh up their options.

You can see how shared decision-making complements an evidence-based approach. Sadly, however, Légaré et al. (2014) noted that even though outcomes appear to be better when patients and clients are involved in decision-making, professionals often do not actively engage with their patients. Légaré et al. (2014) examined interventions to improve adoption of shared decision-making and, despite low-quality evidence, concluded that any intervention that actively targets patients, healthcare professionals or both is better than none.

There are many different activities and decisions that require the use of evidence. Thompson and Stapley (2011) highlight several types of decision:

- Decisions about interventions
- Decisions about which patients or clients will benefit most from an intervention
- Decisions about the best time to intervene
- Decisions about when to deliver information
- Decisions about how to manage a service or care delivery
- Decisions about how to reassure patients and clients.

In the real world of practice, there may be some overlap between these and the types may not be so clear-cut, as you will see from the examples below. In these examples, we describe some of the varied decisions you and your patients/clients may have to make and the different types of evidence available.

Examples of different decisions made by different professionals

Example 1: If you are a midwife, you will regularly provide advice about breastfeeding newborn babies. Some mothers struggle to breastfeed and you might think about suggesting supplementing breastfeeding with bottle-feeding as you have heard other mothers do. You need to check the evidence behind this and ensure that you give the best available advice to new mothers and their babies. In this case, the evidence you need is research that addresses the best form of nutrition for newborn babies.

Example 2: If you are a social worker, you will regularly need to assess risk of depression in clients and you need to be able to suggest effective strategies to support your clients. In this case, the evidence you need is research that addresses the types of interventions that are effective.

Example 3: If you are a surgical nurse, you will regularly need to give an intramuscular injection and you need to know the best site for the injection and the best technique to use. In this case, the evidence you need is evidence that addresses the most appropriate site for giving an injection.

Example 4: If you are an occupational therapist, you will regularly need to discuss fall prevention strategies with clients. In this case, the evidence you need is that which is concerned with effectiveness of different fall prevention strategies.

Example 5: If you are a physiotherapist, you will regularly provide advice to clients with tendonitis and need to know about the effects of exercise versus rest versus alternative strategies. In this case, the evidence you need is that which evaluates the effectiveness of various interventions for tendonitis.

Example 6: If you are working with vulnerable people, you will regularly need to monitor the fluid intake of your clients to ensure they do not suffer from dehydration. You notice that one client is not drinking a lot of fluid. In this case, the evidence you need is about the importance of adequate hydration.

The consequences and implications of your decisions

Accurate clinical judgement and decision-making are vital in diagnosing and delivering safe and effective care (Standing 2015). Thompson et al. (2013: 1720) assert that:

> *Nurses' judgements and decisions have the potential to help health-care systems allocate resources efficiently, promote health gain and patient benefit and prevent harm.*

Thompson et al. (2013) observe that healthcare environments and patients vary and in some instances we will be unsure which interventions are effective. When this is the case, professional and clinical judgement becomes very important. Problems may arise when we do not know which interventions are effective and/or valued by our patients or fail to utilize the available evidence. This will have a negative impact on the overall outcome and cost-effectiveness.

Some decisions will be more important than others. This will depend on the nature of the risk or potential for harm to the patient/client (or the professional) in undertaking or omitting the intervention and the costs involved.

The box above provides examples of where the decisions to be made have serious implications. If mothers are not properly supported to breast-feed, the longer-term health of their babies may be compromised (Lessen and Kavanagh 2015). If the occupational therapist does not provide appropriate advice regarding falls prevention, a patient or client may have a serious accident (Nagayama et al. 2015). Even if a decision does not appear life-threatening – for example, the management of tendonitis – these conditions can have a serious impact on the quality of the patient's life.

Consider activities/interventions in your own professional practice. Which of these carry a higher risk? Are these activities or interventions based on evidence?

Below, we provide an example of a decision that most people would probably consider to have few implications, together with examples of decisions that most people would likely consider to be more serious.

Examples from practice

Example 1: A young man asks your advice regarding his eczema. He has dry skin and intense itching and asks if he should use an emollient cream, and if so, which one? You take a minute to check if there have been any systematic reviews on the use of emollient creams in eczema. Van Zuuren et al. (2017: 3) conclude that 'Moisturisers are safe, prevent flares, prolong time to flare, reduce the amount of topical corticosteroids needed to achieve similar reductions in disease severity, and that topical active treatment is more effective when used in combination with moisturisers.' You offer the young man the plain language summary of the review so he can be involved in the decision of what to use.

Example 2: A person in a health or social care setting notices that not all staff are washing their hands between seeing patients or clients that they care for. The decision of the healthcare provider to omit hand hygiene is high-risk. There is evidence that all health and social care practitioners should thoroughly decontaminate their hands between episodes of patient/client contact. Hand cleansing is probably the most important strategy for infection control, something that has been highlighted by many large systematic reviews (e.g. Jefferson et al. 2011). This is an inexpensive task but a highly effective one that can have serious consequences if not followed meticulously. Thus, failure to follow this evidence-based practice would be very difficult, if not impossible, to justify.

Hand washing, of course, is important on a global scale. Imagine your colleague is planning on volunteering in a low- or middle-income country (LMIC) and you are trying to identify what evidence might be most informative for her trip. You find a systematic review (Ejemot-Nwadiaro et al. 2015) on the promotion of hand washing in the prevention of diarrhoea that you think will be relevant. It concludes that: 'Hand washing promotion probably reduces diarrhoea episodes in both child daycare centres in high-income countries and among communities living in LMICs by about 30%.'

Example 3: Complex decision-making was the focus of a systematic review by Massey et al. (2017), who investigated how quickly professionals respond to the deteriorating patient. They found that 'ward nurses were anxious about making the wrong decision and looking foolish or stupid, and these feelings delayed response to patient deterioration' (p. 19). The authors concluded that "issues involved in timely recognition of and response to clinical deterioration remain complex, yet patient safety relies on nurses' timely assessments and actions' (p. 1).

Importance and urgency in decision-making

We have shown that some decisions might be more significant than others and that the decision to respond to a patient's or client's request for information about the use of moisturizers for eczema might be less important or urgent than other decisions you make, such as washing your hands or responding to a deteriorating patient. Although it is sometimes difficult to assess the urgency or importance of decisions we make, the more aware we are of and informed about key evidence, the more likely we are to make an informed EBP decision when it is especially important or urgent.

The greater the risk to the patient/client or likelihood of harm, the more important it is that your practice is based on evidence. However, you ought to consider the evidence base behind all of the practice you undertake. If there is good evidence available about the decision you need to make, you should use this in your decision-making if your professional judgement, circumstances, patient preference, and resources permit.

Finding out that there is no available research evidence, *rather than assuming that there is none, is valuable information you can use to justify why you need to use other forms of evidence.*

The types of evidence we need to make different decisions

Just as there are many types of decisions that you make on a daily basis, there are also many types of evidence you will use to underpin those decisions.

 In general terms, you should adopt the most appropriate interventions and be able to justify them with reference to the most appropriate evidence.

Evidence will often be from **primary research** or better still **reviews of research** (often referred to as systematic reviews), examples of which we have already mentioned. Research allows direct observation of the effects of interventions and care procedures on patients/clients and, in the case of qualitative research, provides us with insight so that we may more fully understand a situation or service users' experiences.

Many health and social care professionals have busy work lives and will have limited time available to access systematic literature reviews or individual research studies. For this reason, summaries of evidence are available, including international, national, and local **policies, guidelines, clinical knowledge summaries**, and **care pathways.** Whatever your profession or country of practice, it is worth searching for specific websites that draw together **evidence summaries** for particular topics (see the Appendix for useful websites). This approach is preferred to the use of search engines such as Google. We discuss practical examples of accessing evidence further in Chapters 5 and 7.

If there is no research evidence, you might draw on established scientific information such as anatomy, physiology, pathophysiology, microbiology, pharmacokinetics/pharmacodynamics, biomechanics, and so on, and use this evidence to make reasoned deductions about what you need to know. In addition, by adopting a more holistic and creative approach in the health and social care professions, you can draw on a wider range of perspectives, including those of sociology, psychology, epidemiology, anthropology, the arts, and technology to help make decisions. Sometimes you will not look to research to make your decision but will need different evidence, for example, professional codes of conduct, legal precedents or ethical principles.

Whether such codes, laws, and ethics can be considered 'evidence' is a matter of debate. However, they certainly contribute to our ability to provide a clear rationale for our practice. Your practice would not withstand scrutiny if you relied on unprofessional, unlawful or unethical practices.

Professional practice in all areas can be very complex. Standing (2014) argues that there are likely to be a range of factors that you need to consider when making a decision, and these will depend on the complexity of the decision and the time available. Standing has developed a continuum that illustrates how, if you have sufficient time and the appropriate resources, you will be able to make a considered and rational decision, fully informed by relevant evidence. If you have less time and you are responding to an individual, local patient/client crisis, your decision is likely to be more reactionary. This is where the use of policy and guidelines is useful, as they can provide evidence-based guidance in circumstances where you need to make a quick decision. You are also likely to draw on **patient/ client opinion**, your own intuition and **reflective judgement**, and the **expertise of others** when you make a complex decision in a specific context – particularly where there are time pressures. These constitute the **clinical** or **professional judgement** component of evidence-based practice. However, if you experience the same situation repeatedly in your practice, you should invest time accessing the best available evidence so you are well informed when you need to make a fast decision. You should not use lack of time in the moment as an excuse for not keeping up to date.

Standing (2014) argues that the role of the decision-maker is to be professionally accountable for assessing patient/clients' needs using **appropriate sources of information** and planning interventions that address their problems. In the examples we give throughout this chapter, we will emphasize that there are many different types of evidence that you can draw on in your professional decision-making.

Let's have a look at some of the decisions you are likely to be faced with in everyday practice. You will see that the type of evidence needed to make these decisions comes, from a range of sources, not just research evidence.

Examples of decisions and the type of evidence they require

Decision 1: My patient/client has been a long-term heavy alcohol user and wants to self-discharge against the judgement of staff. What should I do?

*Evidence you need to help you make a decision – you would need to adopt relevant **legal and ethical principles** regarding the rights of the patient/client to self-discharge and the duty owed to him by the health or* *social care practitioner. Local **policy** may also guide this decision. You may also use **professional judgement** and **prior experience** in exploring with him the options for his care. You might refer to your **professional body standards** too.*

Decision 2: A mature student on placement has considerable personal issues and they don't appear to be coping well. How shall I handle it?

Evidence you need to help you make decision – you would need to find out the university policy on supporting students, you may seek the views of your colleagues or the expert opinion of a tutor. You may also use your intuition and experience to help you respond to particular issues. You could find qualitative research that explores the mature student experience of placements.

Decision 3: My patient/client has asked me about the use of acupuncture as a pain-relieving agent. What should I advise?

Evidence you need to help you make a decision – to answer any questions about the effectiveness of an intervention, you would need to find research, ideally in the form of systematic reviews or randomized controlled trials that have looked specifically at the issue in question (we will discuss what randomized controlled trials are and why they are needed later).

Decision 4: A client with depression wants to have more access to his children. How can I best support him?

Evidence you need to help you make a decision – you would need to explore the client's rights as a father from a legal perspective, and the implications of his depression on his ability to care for his children. You might use qualitative research about the experiences of those with depression coping with parenthood.

Decision 5: I want to know if I should expel the air bubble in a syringe of Fragmin (a drug to reduce the incidence of deep vein thrombosis) before administering an injection. What should I do?

Evidence you need to help you make a decision – you would search to see if there is any research evidence, but in the absence of any you should consult the most recent instructions on the manufacturer's website [http://www.pfizer.ca/products/fragmin-dalteparin-sodium-injection] for any rationale given. In this case, the air bubble ensures the full dose of the drug is given.

Decision 6: My patient/client with cognitive impairment seems restless and I am wondering if I should ensure they are given their 'as required' pain medication?

> *Evidence you need to help you make a decision* – *you could search a health or social care database for a review of studies on 'pain assessment in cognitively impaired adults' (we discuss searching in Chapter 5). You may find validated assessment tools or advice on how best to assess this client group (e.g. Corbett et al. 2014). You could discuss the behaviour with family/carers to see if it is indicative of pain. You could use other physiological measurements such as pulse and blood pressure recordings to assess the individual. You might locate studies that report that pain is generally under-assessed and under-treated in those with cognitive impairment.*

You can see from these examples that we make decisions in a wide variety of contexts and that a variety of forms of evidence are needed. When you are looking for evidence on your topic, 'one size' really does not fit all. If anyone tells you that you 'always need research evidence' to answer your question, this would be misleading – you need the most relevant information to answer your question. This is often research but as we have seen in the previous examples, it might come from another source, such as a policy document or legal or ethical principles. In a busy professional context, when you are managing complex situations, you may find that there is no easy fit between the evidence and the environment you are working in. The type of evidence you need depends on the decision you have to make and you need to think carefully about this to work out the best type of evidence.

You should not use 'lack of time' as a reason to avoid seeking out the best available evidence, as you have a professional responsibility to keep yourself up to date.

When you search for evidence to use in your practice, it is sometimes referred to as practising in an 'evidence-informed way'. The difficulty is that no one can tell you what type of evidence you need in a given set of circumstances – you need to base this on your own judgement.

Getting started: defining your question or decision

You should start by clarifying and narrowing down the question or exact decision you need to make. The first thing you need to do is to **define a question/refine the decision** that identifies what you need to know. This is important because unless you are focused, you will be swamped with too much irrelevant information. We will discuss a more structured way of forming a question in much more detail in Chapter 5.

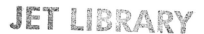

LIBRARY, UNIVERSITY OF CHESTER

Example from practice

A friend asks about anti-malarial tablets, as she is about to go on a foreign adventure. Where would you start?

First, you need to clarify exactly what your friend wants to know. What exactly are you being asked? Is your friend concerned about . . .

- The effectiveness of the various types of anti-malarial tablets on the market?
- The health and environmental effects of the tablets?
- The cost?
- The best time to travel to avoid mosquitoes?
- People's experiences of using the various tablets?

If you are unable to identify exactly what your friend wants to know, you will not be able to find the appropriate evidence to advise them in a meaningful way. You might find out which anti-malarial is most effective when what they really want to know is which is the cheapest. The information you do find is likely to be of limited use if it doesn't address what your friend wants to know.

The message is clear – even when you have a rather broad topic, you need to know what the question is before you begin to look for the right type of evidence.

 Select a topic from your own professional practice and think about how you might address several different questions, each with a different focus.

If you are looking for evidence about the effectiveness of anti-malarial tablets, this evidence will not be the same as what you would search for when looking for evidence about the experiences of those who have used different tablets.

What kinds of evidence are there?

There are many decisions you will make and many different kinds of evidence that will assist your decision-making. As we said previously, evidence comes in many forms. What would be considered weak evidence for one decision would be stronger evidence for another decision. Consider again the six decisions, described earlier, that required evidence. Different types of evidence were needed to assist with decision-making – professional, legal and ethical principles, policy, guidelines and research evidence, together with clinical and professional judgement. It is important to identify the type of evidence you need.

Anecdotal evidence

You are probably familiar with the term **anecdotal evidence**. This is generally a weaker form of evidence for all types of decisions for the reasons outlined below. However, if no other evidence is available, then anecdotal evidence will have to do.

In health and social care, **anecdotal evidence** can be drawn from:

- experience – something you tried before that worked;
- a colleague or practice assessor/mentor who says, 'we've always done it like this';
- discussion papers, opinion articles or editorials;
- experts (consultants, specialist practitioners, other colleagues; although their opinion is very likely to be informed by evidence, do not assume this to be the case!).

In principle, you should be aware that the quality of evidence provided by anecdotal information – even if it is based on expert opinion – is generally weaker than that which is provided by research or reviews of research. Remember that if you do not ask for the evidence that lies behind the advice you are given, you might be practising using anecdotal evidence only and your practice would not stand up to scrutiny. However, published material that does not report research findings can still be useful in the absence of research.

Example from practice

Imagine you are trying to train your dog. He is not an easy dog to train – he is somewhat feisty and pulls on the lead. You experiment with a few choker collars that pull tighter around his neck when he pulls and relaxes when he walks to heel. Your aim is to find out which one he responds to best. You find one that seems to be a good fit and deters him from pulling on the lead. Here you have some evidence about which choker lead works best – at least for you and your dog. This is anecdotal evidence based on trial and error and is the type of evidence that people have gathered and used over the generations. Indeed, a lot of health and social care has been based on anecdotal evidence in the absence of hard evidence being available. Now imagine that you have hundreds of dogs at a Guide Dog training centre and you need to know which lead works the best. **Here the stakes are higher for many reasons:**

- The effective training of the dogs is even more important because of the role they are to perform.
- There are cost implications, as each dog to be trained will require a lead.
- The time taken to train the dog also has cost implications.

If you were a recipient of a guide dog or a donator to the charitable organization Guide Dogs for the Blind, you would want to know that the best lead was being used to train the dogs. In this instance, the anecdotal evidence gleaned from the experience of one person attempting to train his dog would not be sufficient. You would want more robust evidence upon which to base your choice of dog lead.

This scenario can be transferred to any health or social care settings in which the stakes are high. There are limited resources and patients/clients expect and have a right to receive optimum care. We cannot afford to get it wrong. Anecdotal evidence – or trial and error – is clearly not enough. We cannot afford to base practice on insubstantial evidence that does not stand up to scrutiny. However, with discretion, anecdotal information can be useful in the following ways:

- It can contribute to your professional judgement.
- It can be used to set the context/give background information.
- It can be used to identify what is common practice when there is little or no other conclusive evidence.

In the same way that the Guide Dog trainer needs good evidence about the effectiveness of the different dog leads that are available, so the health and social care provider needs good evidence about the effectiveness of the care they deliver. With the availability of systematic and rigorous research studies, we now have more robust evidence upon which to base our practice.

In Chapter 2, we discussed how the 'information revolution', the Internet, and social media can lead to information overload, and how it can be difficult to verify this information. This can mean that anecdotal evidence receives more coverage than might appear reasonable given the quality of the information provided. Van der Linden describes how 'expert consensus is easily undermined by anecdotal evidence. Indeed, the so-called "false media balance" frequently distorts the weight of evidence on vaccine safety' (2016: 119).

In contrast, Kailasam and Samuels (2015) argue that so-called anecdotal evidence may have some value. They present a case study of a patient who announced intending committing suicide on Facebook. The authors note that social networking sites are sources of real-time information that could aid in suicide prevention, and consider that social media may present opportunities for early intervention.

Research evidence

So, if we need to move away from anecdotal evidence, what do we move towards? As the earlier examples of decisions and evidence types illustrate, different forms of evidence will inform your practice and decision-making. Legal rulings and ethical argument are examples of this. In most instances, however, research evidence will underpin your practice decisions.

It is important that we use the right evidence for the question we want to answer.

In Chapter 4, we discuss the different types of research in detail. For the flow of argument here, however, we discuss some more general principles and ideas. The following examples illustrate that different types of research are needed to answer different questions and that 'one size does not fit all'. If you find any of the examples unclear, please refer to Chapter 4.

Research about effectiveness or 'does it work?'

If you need to find out about the effectiveness of an intervention or therapy, the only way is to find a study (or review of studies) that has directly compared one thing to another. We call this type of study a 'randomized controlled trial' (RCT). This is because in an RCT there is an intervention group and a control group who do not receive the intervention in question and who act as a direct comparison. Unless you have a direct comparison, you cannot tell if something works or not. Thus, RCTs are the 'gold standard' of evidence you are looking for. However, RCTs will only help you if you are looking at whether a treatment or intervention is effective. If you are not looking at effectiveness, then RCTs will not be the 'gold standard' evidence for your question. If your friend in the example earlier wants to know which anti-malarial tablets are the most effective, you would need to look for an RCT that compared one tablet with one or more others.

 If a manufacturer tells you that their product is effective, but you cannot find an independent RCT to back this up, then you should be wary of that claim!

Research about 'what is it like?'

If you are looking for evidence about people's experiences or feelings, say, users' experience of insect repellents, an RCT is unlikely to help you, unless you find one that compares users' experience of one type against another. Instead, you could look for research reports that explore people's experience, or a review of such research. This is likely to be conducted by asking them about their experience using a qualitative approach and probably in-depth interviews. If your friend who asked you about anti-malarial tablets wants to know about how other people have experienced a particular anti-malarial tablet and the side-effects, you need to look for research that explores patients' experiences of taking malaria tablets.

Research about 'what practitioners or patients/clients actually do?'

If you wish to find out what practitioners or patients/clients do – that is, what really happens in practice (e.g. whether people actually take the anti-malarial tablet when they are in a high-risk area, or whether practitioners wash their hands according to protocol) – you would need to look for studies that directly report on practice. For the first example, whether travellers take their anti-malarial tablets, it might be difficult to discern exactly how many people adhere to a prophylaxis regime without undercover observers, which would clearly be impossible! Instead, those concerned with adherence to the prophylaxis regime against malaria would need to rely on patient reports of adherence to any anti-malarial drug prescribed. This information might be collected in a **questionnaire/survey** or **interview**. There are some occasions, however, when you are able to observe directly what actually happens in practice, for example, in a professional context.

Example from practice

You are concerned about infection in your unit and want to find out about how compliant staff are with hand-washing/hand-rubbing policies. Consider the type of evidence you would you look for. Imagine that you found a questionnaire study that had asked staff at the end of every shift whether they always follow infection control procedures. Consider the answers they are likely to give and whether these would reflect what they *actually* do. How strong would that evidence be? What type of evidence would you look for that would really tell you about staff adherence to infection control policy?

Clearly, the answer is to find **observational studies**, in which a researcher observed whether staff washed their hands – or not – in an everyday context. Any evidence that falls short of this approach would not be very strong. Thus, for this question, the very best type of evidence would be observational studies. Our recall or description of what we do can be different from what we actually do!

Choose an issue/topic in your professional practice and try focusing your question differently to find different types of evidence.

You can see from these examples that it is helpful to be able to 'pinpoint' the type of research you are looking for and that different types of research inform us about different aspects of professional practice and decisions that need to be made. We have argued that research evidence is usually the best evidence to use in our professional practice. When we are thinking about evidence-based practice, we need to ensure that we use the strongest possible evidence to support our practice. If we do not look for strong evidence, we risk being criticized for not using up-to-date, robust evidence. Remember that the nature of evidence in health and social care changes very quickly and what was considered good evidence yesterday can soon become outdated. However, you must also remember that nothing is perfect and you may not always be able to find strong evidence. You should aim to base your practice on the **best available evidence** you can find.

We will now consider how closely research should be related to your professional environment for it to be useful to you. Ideally you will find research that is directly applicable to your area of professional practice but this will not always be the case.

Research that relates directly to your client or patient group

Research that is directly applicable *refers to research evidence that relates directly to the health and social care practice you are involved in.*

In an ideal world, there would be direct evidence to underpin the care you deliver and this evidence would be based on direct observations or studies of people who are similar to those you look after. Also in that ideal world, you would find that the evidence that exists relates directly to your clinical or professional setting so that you can be as sure as possible that it applies to your patient or client.

Examples from practice

Example 1: The process of hand cleansing is the same whichever patients/clients you work with, except of course that for some patients/clients additional infection control precautions apply or the procedures or interventions may be higher or lower risk. Research evidence relating to hand cleansing will be relevant to your practice irrespective of where and when it was undertaken, although of course, you still need to assess the quality of the research undertaken.

Example 2: An example of direct evidence is the impact of shift work on the quality of care. Shift work is an integral component of all practice areas where patients/clients require 24-hour care. Thus, any research that explores quality of care provision and its relationship to shift work is likely to be directly relevant to all disciplines.

More often than not, however, you will come across evidence that does not relate directly to your patient/client or client group or the exact situation you find yourself in. This evidence can still be useful to you as discussed below.

Research conducted with different client or patient groups or in different settings

Much available research will not have been conducted specifically with your patient or client group in mind or in your professional setting but is nonetheless relevant to you. The research might have been carried out on a different group of patients or clients or in a different country, so its relevance and application to your setting might be different. Such research could include:

- Research undertaken with patient or client groups in a related area
- Research that has been undertaken in a laboratory
- Research from other academic disciplines.

Research undertaken with patients or clients groups in a related area

Consider, for example, some research about how information giving reduces anxiety. Let's say that you come across some research that was undertaken with patients/clients in an oncology ward. You are working in general surgery. This evidence will be less directly relevant to your patients/clients and you need to determine the extent to which the research is relevant to you. We will discuss ways of assessing the quality of the evidence later in this book but for now it is important to note that you are likely to have to make a judgement as to the applicability of the evidence you encounter to your professional practice. This is the 'clinical/ professional judgement' component of evidence-based practice we referred to in Chapter 1. However, this research may be relevant to you in some way. This is why we refer to it as indirect evidence.

Alternatively, imagine you are working with deprived children from a particular cultural group in an inner-city area. There is research evidence on the most effective way to promote uptake of day care provision that has been undertaken with a different cultural group but nothing that relates to the particular group of children you are working with. Again, this is where your clinical or professional judgement comes into play. You might find that this is the best available evidence and you need to determine how relevant it is to the group of children you are working with.

You are likely thinking by now that much of the evidence you use in your practice is indirect evidence – that is, even if it was obtained through direct observation or experiments on patient or clients, its focus was not on the practice setting you are working in and therefore the evidence does not apply to your practice directly and you have to make a judgement about its relevance to your practice area. You will find this often to be the case.

Consider why research that was carried out in the USA on the funding of health and social care might not be relevant, yet research carried out there on a therapeutic activity may be so.

The reason may be because the health and social care funding systems are very different between the UK and the USA, but the effectiveness of an intervention will be the same for people with similar issues or problems in the two countries. You need to judge if it is relevant or not.

Research undertaken in a laboratory

You may find that there is no research that is directly applicable or can be applied to your own professional context. Often, there will be insufficient direct or indirect research evidence available that is applicable to the specific question you wish to address. This does not mean that you cannot practise evidence-based practice. You can still find evidence to underpin your practice, even if it is not immediately obvious what information might be relevant to you. Sometimes, the results of research undertaken in a laboratory might be relevant to your professional practice.

Example from practice

Preoperative bathing or showering with an antiseptic skin wash product is a well-accepted procedure for reducing skin bacteria (microflora). It is less clear whether reducing skin microflora leads to fewer surgical site infections (Webster and Osborne 2015). However, this is assumed to be the case and the rationale for asking patients to wash with an antiseptic prior to surgery is based on indirect evidence rather than direct research undertaken in practice.

 Evidence deduced from research undertaken in laboratory conditions may be applied to professional practice.

Your practice can be underpinned by evidence that is deduced from scientific knowledge rather than from research studies that have been carried out on patients/clients directly.

It is often necessary to look further afield for sources that might provide you with an evidence base for your practice. This is because professional practice encompasses a very wide range of activities and will therefore draw on a wide range of sources of evidence to justify practice. Evidence deduced from scientific knowledge is evidence obtained from scientific and social scientific explanations about how things work, but which have not been tested or observed scientifically (empirically) with patient or clients in the practice setting. By scientific knowledge we mean from the hard sciences, such as biology, physiology, and also from social sciences such as sociology and psychology.

Research adopted from other disciplines

We can sometimes use research evidence from other disciplines to provide rationale for our practice. For example, social work practitioners draw widely on research from sociology and psychology, especially regarding attachment behaviours and the critical role of parents in the developing child.

Consider the everyday task of taking a patient's or client's physiological observations. We know from our understanding of physiology that taking the patient/client's vital signs – temperature, pulse, and blood pressure – will provide an indication of the condition of the patient/client. We also know that low blood pressure readings are indicative of haemorrhage. There is, therefore, a physiological rationale for taking a patient's/client's blood pressure following surgery. Yet, to really know how effective this is in the prevention and management of haemorrhage, we would need to observe the effectiveness of this in practice. Recently, there have been concerns that although staff take observations, they are not responding quickly enough to abnormal results and so many institutions have set up guidelines and checklists such as early warning scoring systems as advised by the NICE pathway (NICE 2007/2016).

There are many areas in health and social care that require us to draw on knowledge outside of our immediate specialty. For example, Van El et al. (2013) recommend that professionals engage with the impact of genetics in their day-to-day practice.

All our professions rely on knowledge from many different disciplines, including sociology, psychology, and pharmacology.

You are likely to find that your own area of practice is informed by a wide variety of disciplines and that research from within these disciplines will be relevant to your practice. You will use these to develop an understanding of the evidence base behind many of the activities you undertake. You might therefore need to think and search quite broadly to find evidence to justify and inform your practice.

What other specialist disciplines are predominant in informing your professional practice?

Once you have done this, you may be able to identify the direct and indirect sources of research evidence that influence your practice.

The disciplines from which we might draw evidence include:

Physiology and pathophysiology, medicine (many branches), pharmacology, sociology, immunology, ethics, law, dietetics, radiology, epidemiology, cytology, microbiology, gerontology, anatomy, psychiatry, psychology, podiatry, art, politics, philosophy, theology, technology.

What other 'evidence' is out there?

You will not always find direct or indirect research information on your topic – either a literature review or individual pieces of research. Imagine a line where traditional practices and ritual are at one end and a fully evidence-based approach at the other:

Ritualistic practice   Evidence-based practice

←——————————————————————————————→

You would like to think that the majority of health and social care interventions fall at the evidence-based end of the continuum. Unfortunately, however, there are still many areas where there is a lack of research, as can be seen from a number of Cochrane and Campbell reviews. In some of these cases, the quality of research is not good enough to draw conclusions from and so more or higher quality research is needed.

There is no research evidence or only evidence of poor quality

As we discussed in Chapter 2, sometimes you may not find any research-based information, or you might not be in a position to identify the best possible evidence. As we suggested earlier in this chapter, if this is the case, you will need to rely on other sources of knowledge and evidence, such as experience and advice from colleagues. Be aware that, depending on the task, time issue or problem, these may provide a weaker source of evidence.

Always try to avoid sources of information where the author, the credibility of the information or date of publication is unclear, such as those you might come across casually on the Internet.

Think about your own everyday practice. How much of it do you think should and can be based on actual high-quality evidence?

The best evidence to look for is:

- **Systematic literature reviews:** probably the most important single source of evidence, as we will explain in the next chapter.
- **Research papers:** remember that all topics are diverse and you need to find a paper that looks at your particular research interest – that is, a research paper that explores whether a new intervention is acceptable to patients or clients is very different from one that explores whether it works! Make sure the aim of the research paper reflects your own information needs.

Evidence to be cautious of includes:

- **Evidence obtained through broad use of search engines:** beware of sources retrieved through random search engine searches such as **Google.**
- **Unknown websites:** websites can be useful. We will discuss these in Chapter 6. However, it is vital that you assess the sources upon which the website is based.
- **Public/charitable websites:** be aware that information posted here may have no clearly named author, may have been summarized by a non-health or social care professional, and may have been over-simplified or even have an agenda. These sites can provide some useful overview information but do try and find an original source and author for the information claims made.
- **Wikipedia:** the information on Wikipedia is placed there or edited by members of the public. While it is sometimes useful for providing explanations or key authors names, it should not be relied upon. It may help you identify key search terms to use on more reliable databases.

- **One single piece of non-research-based evidence that makes a claim about practice:** this might be an opinion piece or practice paper found in a professional journal. We will consider how to judge the quality of the evidence that you find in Chapter 6 but the point we would like to make here is that one piece of literature, even research, is rarely enough for you to base your practice on.
- **What your colleagues, practice assessors/mentors say:** although much learning occurs through the sharing of information between those who are more experienced and those with less experience or skill, you should adopt a critical approach to accepting this information as evidence – especially when the source of their knowledge cannot be stated.

In summary

Every time you need to make a decision, you need to consider the evidence base you can draw on to make that decision. Asking your colleague or practice assessor/mentor is not enough! Research-based evidence should normally be drawn on in the first instance unless the situation requires another form of evidence such as a legal ruling or ethical argument. If no research evidence is available, then you will need to draw on weaker evidence. It is important to recognize how strong the evidence is that you draw upon, as this reflects how much confidence you can have in the evidence you use.

Key points

1 Every time you need to make a decision, consider what evidence you need to base your decision upon.
2 There are many different types of decision and many different types of evidence to use.
3 You will **normally** use research evidence in the first instance.
4 At other times you will need a different rationale – for example, ethical principles or legal guidance.
5 Some research will be directly relevant to your question; other research will be less relevant.
6 You might also use physiological, psychological, sociological or pharmacological evidence or, where relevant, theory, reflective judgement or intuition.
7 Policy and guidelines should be based on research evidence.
8 Use anecdotal evidence as a last resort.

Quiz questions

1 What factors do you need to consider regarding (or in relation to) the potential consequences of your decision-making?
2 When is it appropriate to use different types of evidence?
3 What types of evidence should you be wary of?

4 What are the different types of research and how do they help us to answer different questions?

In the previous chapter, we provided a broad overview of the decisions you will make as a health or social care professional and the different kinds of evidence you will draw on. In this chapter, we will consider:

* The different types of research in detail and other evidence that you might find
* How the question you want to answer influences the type of evidence you look for.

We acknowledge that evidence-based practice does not necessarily mean that you will always be using research evidence, although this will often be the case. Therefore, given that research can be hard to understand, we devote this chapter to summarizing the types of research evidence you are likely to encounter. We advise that you dip in and out of this chapter regarding specific research methods when you need to find out about them.

How do I recognize research?

Research is generally recognizable by the way it is presented. Research follows a clear structure that is usually described in the **abstract** (a paragraph that usually appears on on the first page of a paper).

Research is a systematic activity that follows a clear process.

The research process:

1 Identify a clinical or professional problem
2 Search the literature (in case your problem has a known solution)
3 Critically read the research (to identify limitations or gaps)
4 Form a **research question** or state a **hypothesis** (statement) or aims
5 Consider any relevant ethical issues or permissions
6 Decide on an appropriate research method
7 Collect the data
8 Analyse the data
9 Interpret the results
10 Publish and disseminate the findings.

It is important to recognize this process from the start. Research normally begins with a question, hypothesis or clear statement of aims, which is followed by a description of how the study was conducted (usually called the methods or methodology), then the results/findings and conclusion. The research methods outlined below are just some of those that you might encounter. It is important that you become familiar with the different approaches to research design so that you can judge its relevance and quality. We will discuss this in greater detail in Chapter 6.

 Brainstorm any research methods that you have heard of.

The research evidence you might come across can be classified as follows:

• **Systematic reviews or good quality literature reviews**
• **Quantitative research** (sometimes called **primary research**), of which there are many different types but classified into:
  o **Experimental methods** (where an intervention is given to one group and not to another and the outcome is observed), e.g. randomized controlled trials (RCTs) and quasi-experiments
  o **Non-experimental methods** (where no intervention is given and populations are observed and compared with a control group), e.g. cohort and case controlled studies, cross-sectional studies, numerical reporting or scales used in questionnaires/surveys
• **Qualitative research** (sometimes called **primary research**), of which there are many different approaches, including:
  o Grounded theory
  o Phenomenology
  o Ethnography
  o Action research

Systematic reviews, rapid reviews, and good quality literature reviews

Systematic reviews

 See this useful video from Cochrane: 'What are systematic reviews?' [http://www.cochrane.org/what-is-cochrane-evidence].

Note that in the settings section you can select subtitles for different languages.

Systematic reviews and good quality literature reviews are very useful because they aim to summarize **all** the available literature on a topic, whether qualitative or quantitative. A literature review might be referred to as a **systematic review**, and this is the name given to a very detailed review of literature on a topic. The term 'systematic review' comes from the **Cochrane** and **Campbell Collaborations**, organizations that commission literature reviews within health and social care. The Cochrane Collaboration focuses on 'producing reviews that summarize the best available evidence generated through research to inform decisions about health' [see http://uk.cochrane.org/about-us], while the Campbell Collaboration's mission statement states that it 'promotes positive social and economic change through the production and use of systematic reviews and other evidence synthesis for evidence-based policy and practice' [see https://www.campbellcollaboration.org/about-campbell/vision-mission-and-principle.html]. So, if you come across a systematic review, you can be fairly sure you have found a good quality review. Systematic literature reviews are referred to as original empirical research because they review, evaluate, and synthesize all the available primary data, which can be either quantitative or qualitative.

Cochrane is available in different languages [see http://www.cochrane.org/translation]. These include: English, Deutsch, Español, Français, Hrvatski, 日本語, 한국어, Bahasa Malaysia, Polski, Português, Русский, 简体中文, 繁體中文.

A systematic review aims to identify and track down all the available literature on a topic with clear explanation of the methods taken by the reviewers.

Systematic reviews can be found on both health and social care topics and using any type of research. However, reviews published by the Cochrane and Campbell Collaborations focus on the effectiveness of care and treatment interventions.

The Cochrane Library can be searched by topic or by Cochrane specialist group, such as Public Health, Childhood Cancer, Developmental, Psychosocial, Learning Problems [available at: http://www.cochranelibrary.com/cochrane-database-of-systematic-reviews/index.html].

The Campbell Library has similar search strategies [available at: https://www.campbellcollaboration.org/better-evidence.html].

Both the Cochrane and Campbell Collaborations have a plain English summary of the reviews to help you understand complex medical or sociological terms or concepts.

Rapid reviews

The detailed and comprehensive methods used by those doing a systematic review are well established. However, it is also recognized that doing a systematic review is resource-intensive and takes a long time (Abou-Setta et al. 2016). As a solution, the concept of a rapid review has been suggested as a means of providing information for decision-making within a shorter timeframe. Featherstone et al. (2015) carried out a systematic literature search to explore the concept of rapid reviews and found 12 papers. They concluded that the methods and approaches used for rapid reviews vary greatly, as do the definitions. However, they concluded that they do have the potential to answer narrow questions of efficacy or effectiveness in a shorter time, and using fewer resources than a standard systematic review.

Abou-Setta et al. (2016) also found that rapid reviews drew similar conclusions to those of systematic reviews, but they concluded that there is currently a lack of evidence about the overall validity of rapid reviews. In view of this, the Cochrane Collaboration have set up a group to inform the development of this methodology [see http://methods.cochrane.org/news/rapid-reviews methods group]

Rapid synthesis of available evidence can be useful in the absence of high quality systematic reviews or when a decision is needed quickly. For example, Best Evidence Topics (BestBets, n.d.) use a systematic approach and have a searchable database [see http://www.bestbets.org/].

In addition to systematic and rapid reviews, there are other less detailed reviews that you might come across. You may find a **literature review** (*without* the prefix 'systematic'). However, if the word 'systematic' is not found in the title, you might still have a high-quality review – but you need to take a look at how the review was undertaken, which will allow you to form a judgement about the quality of the review.

How can I recognize a systematic review or a good literature review when I come across one?

Most obviously, of course, the title of the review will usually contain the words 'literature review' or 'systematic review'. However, the review itself will contain a written **method**; this is often clearly stated in the abstract (on the first page of the article) as well as in a dedicated section that describes how the literature has been systematically searched for and how the authors assessed the quality of the papers they included. If this is not explained, it is difficult to determine if the review has been carried out in a comprehensive manner and therefore how thorough it is. In reviews today, you would expect to see a PRISMA (Preferred Reporting Items for Systematic reviews and Meta-Analyses) statement, which consists of a 27-item checklist and a four-phase flow diagram. The aim of the PRISMA statement is to document a clear search process and hence help authors improve the reporting of the search processes undertaken in systematic reviews and meta-analyses (Moher et al. 2009).

Systematic reviews are often undertaken with quantitative research, especially randomized controlled trials, but they can also be done with qualitative research and studies of mixed methods.

Be wary of papers described as a 'literature review' or 'review' but which do not tell you how the review was compiled. The authors may have 'cherry picked' what they wanted to include or ignored large areas of literature. There are lots of these 'review' papers in the literature and many are extremely useful, written by experts. However, it is important to remember that unless the authors tell you how they searched and appraised the literature they included, it is not possible to tell whether the paper presents a balanced argument.

Example

Linus Pauling (1986), a highly accredited scientist, wrote a book entitled *How to Live Longer and Feel Better*, in which he quoted from a selection of articles that supported his opinion that vitamin C contains properties that are effective against the common cold. This book makes an interesting and convincing read. At first glance, you might think it to be a comprehensive literature review, but no methodology was included in the book and, much later on, when a systematic review was undertaken of all the evidence surrounding the effectiveness of vitamin C (Knipschild 1994), no evidence of the effectiveness of vitamin C was identified. This illustrates how a non-systematic review can be misleading.

A systematic review or good quality literature review will be written up in the same manner as a research article. It should include:

- A clear research/review question
- Aims and objectives
- A methods section outlining how the review was undertaken
- A results/findings section
- A discussion and conclusion.

If a review you find does not contain a research question, aims and objectives, methods, results, discussion and conclusion, then it is unlikely to be a thorough, systematic literature review.

Why are reviews so useful?

Literature reviews are important because they seek to:

- Summarize the literature that is available on any one topic.
- Prevent one 'high-profile' piece of information having too much influence.
- Present an analysis of the available literature so that the reader does not have to access each individual research report included in the review.

A systematic review is like having all the pieces of a jigsaw puzzle to hand instead of just a few, thus allowing you to see the full picture (of the evidence).

Often, a piece of research published this month contradicts the findings of a piece of research published last month. For example, one week we are told that alcohol has certain health benefits, then the next week we are told that it is harmful. There is often confusion – people are trying to make sense of the differing messages conveyed and wonder why the results can vary so much. This can be a result of:

- Looking at the results of a study in isolation rather than in the context of others.
- Media portrayal of the research in which a complex set of results is reduced to a simplified message.
- Not acknowledging that there are many aspects of health and social care, e.g. alcohol might have a positive effect on one aspect and a damaging effect on another.

There are many reasons for this:

- The research might have been undertaken in a specific area of practice or with a specific group of people or sample, and is not applicable (or generalizable) to other areas/groups.
- There might be flaws in the research design that affect its overall usefulness.
- Sometimes a hesitant claim or inconclusive result will be interpreted as a certainty.

Therefore, when you read research or a report that seems to conflict with something you read the previous week, it is important to consider the merits of each and to remember that no single piece of research should be viewed in isolation.

Try identifying examples of conflicting information in your own practice and then consider how much better it would be if all the information was brought together so you could see the bigger picture.

Systematic reviews and literature reviews put the evidence into context. They prevent one piece of evidence having excessive influence. One isolated piece of literature can be misleading. Take the story of the measles, mumps, and rubella (MMR) vaccine. In 1998, Wakefield and colleagues published an article in *The Lancet* suggesting that there was a possibility of a link between the MMR vaccination, autism, and bowel disorders. This article was based on a small case study of twelve children who had attended the hospital at which Wakefield worked. Each had the conditions above and also had had the vaccination. Wakefield stated that there were possible environmental triggers to the development of autism in these children, but without a control group and with a very small sample, this could not be confirmed.

The paper published by Wakefield provided one piece of a very large jigsaw. At that time, there were no other data pointing to a potential link between autism and bowel disease. However, as time went on, many further studies were undertaken, none of which confirmed any evidence of a link. It is quite clear from the basic facts in the original paper that the evidence presented is not very strong. Indeed, *The Lancet* subsequently retracted the paper and the debate surrounding the case continues unabated (Kmietowicz 2012; Mellis 2015). However, seen in isolation, this report sparked alarm in both media and medical circles alike. Systematic reviews and literature reviews help to shed new light on things.

The MMR controversy provides one clear example as to why it is important to review all the evidence together and how one piece of information can give a misleading picture. Without the comprehensive review of the literature that followed, the concerns expressed in Wakefield's paper could not have been refuted. There are many similar examples in the literature. For example, in a Cochrane review by Farley et al. (2012), the role of a drug used to facilitate weight loss was reviewed. It had been previously thought that the use of drugs played only a minor role in weight loss facilitation programmes. On reviewing the available literature in a systematic way, the role of these drugs was found to be greater than had originally been thought.

Key features of a systematic review or good quality literature review

The following highlights the main features of a systematic review or a detailed literature review. As an example, at points throughout we draw on a published systematic review by Graham et al. (2016).
Reviewers should:

- Identify a clearly *pre-defined question.*
- Undertake a *comprehensive* and *thorough search* for relevant literature, and demonstrate how this was done.
- Develop *inclusion* and *exclusion criteria* in order to assess which information should be included in the review to ensure that only those papers that are relevant to the question(s) are included.
- Search for *hard-to-find* articles, including ones that have not been published or not yet accepted for publication. This is because there is evidence that studies showing a positive result are more likely to be published – hence using only published studies could bias the result of the review.
- State whether the papers have been appraised and *graded* according to *pre-defined criteria*, and also whether only papers with a high grade are included in the review.
- Synthesize or collate the results and do a meta-analysis where possible (if it is a quantitative review and the studies are similar).
- Discuss any limitations (potential weaknesses) of the study.
- Report the study clearly.

See also 'What makes a good systematic review' (Centre for Evidence Based Information (CEBI), University of Oxford, n.d.) [available at: https://www.cebi.ox.ac.uk/for-practitioners/what-is-good-evidence/what-makes-a-good-systematic-review.html].

Example

Graham et al. (2016) undertook a systematic review to determine whether interventions to enhance employment prospects are effective. The Campbell Collaboration, a publisher of reviews in social care, published the review by Graham and colleagues. Given the importance of reviews to an evidence-based approach, we will discuss this example in detail. The question addressed by the review is the effectiveness of employment interventions on the return to work of those who have experienced a traumatic brain injury. This is clearly an important topic, as it is crucial to target interventions where they will be most beneficial. In order to find as many relevant studies as possible, Graham et al. undertook a very detailed search strategy of many electronic databases. This included searching for unpublished and grey literature and examining the reference lists of the included papers.

Another qualitative review on the barriers and facilitators related to the implementation of surgical safety checklists was undertaken by Bergs et al. (2015), who searched just one database, but the authors clearly outlined their search methods.

Once the reviewers have identified the range of literature to be included in the review, the next step is to assess the quality of the literature to see if it is good enough to help answer the question – using poor quality evidence may provide a misleading picture.

Researchers should *critique* (or judge) the quality of the selected papers to assess the quality of the research identified. Studies that do not meet the inclusion and quality criteria ought to be excluded from the review. This is to ensure that only high-quality and relevant papers are included.

There are various approaches to critically appraising papers for inclusion in a review. Graham et al. identified the risk of bias for each paper included and referred to this in their on-going analysis:

Cochrane's risk of bias tool (i.e., sequence generation, allocation concealment, blinding, incomplete data, and selective outcome reporting; Higgins and Altman 2008), along with study design, review status, type of publication, and control group, were used to assess the chance of bias. Each factor was coded as low risk, high risk, or unclear/unknown for each potential study to be included.

(Graham et al. 2016: 27)

Finally, reviewers should *combine* the findings of all the papers that are used using a systematic approach. This enables new insights to be drawn from the summary of the papers that were not available before. A **meta-analysis** is a way of combining the statistical results of different studies using statistics so that it is possible to merge the results of several studies, rather than having many different results from smaller studies. It is not always possible to undertake a meta-analysis, as demonstrated by Graham and colleagues, and where a review does not contain statistical results, a meta-analysis is not possible and a **thematic analysis** is undertaken instead.

Graham et al. did not use meta-analysis because they did not have enough studies to make a meaningful combination of the results:

Three RCTs comparing two intervention groups were found . . . A meta-analysis was not performed due to the small number of included studies. Although all study interventions led to competitive employment, no one intervention was identified as more effective than the rest. A larger sample of studies is needed to provide a conclusive determination.

(Graham et al. 2016: 41)

In their qualitative review, Bergs et al. (2015) used thematic analysis and argued that the strength of this approach is that it can enable conclusions to be drawn on the basis of common elements of the included qualitative studies.

It is important to remember that a meta-analysis can only be carried out if all the research papers in the literature review have been undertaken in a similar way. And, as meta-analysis is a statistical technique, it can only be undertaken on papers that have their results presented as statistics. Where a meta-analysis has been undertaken, the results are often presented using a **forest plot**, in which the average result of each study is plotted so that it can be easily compared with other studies. As we will see later in this chapter, not all research papers present their results as statistics and for those that do not, it is not possible to undertake a meta-analysis. For these more **qualitative papers**, it is possible to combine the results, which may be presented as themes, using a process known as **meta-synthesis** or **meta-study**.

Graham et al. found no strong evidence to indicate that interventions to enhance employment were beneficial and concluded in the results of the study that:

In summary, this systematic report offers tentative findings for military interventions and samples, but, as with other systematic reviews, offers no conclusive findings on the most effective intervention.

(Graham et al. 2016: 48)

Consult http://www.cochranelibrary.com/ or https://www.campbellcollaboration.
org/library.html for a review relating to a topic relevant to your own
professional practice See if it has all the components of a systematic
review we have described.

Literature reviews (using less detailed approaches)

If you come across a literature review that is not specifically called a
systematic review, this can still be a useful find if the review has been
carried out in a systematic manner, even when not in the detail required
by the Cochrane Library or Campbell Collaboration. What is important
is to look at the way in which the review was undertaken, and make
sure you can see a clear question, search strategy, and a method of
appraisal.

If you come across what you think might be a literature review but
which has no clearly defined method or systematic approach, you should
be less confident in the results of this review. These are sometimes
referred to as **narrative** or **descriptive reviews**. In principle, you should
be cautious about a literature review that:

- has no focused research question;
- has no detailed and complete search strategy;
- has no clear method of appraisal or synthesis of literature;
- is not easily **repeatable**.

As a consequence of the above, the conclusions drawn are likely to be
inaccurate. These reviews are likely to have a number of biases, including
the personal bias of the author(s), as was evident in Linus Pauling's (1986)
book mentioned previously. If there is no clear method section, there is
likely to be a **selection bias** of included material and conclusions, which
cannot be easily verified and may therefore be misleading.

Many research papers provide an initial, brief literature review. This is
usually an overview of previous and current research and helps to
explain why the study is being undertaken.

In summary, literature reviews are very useful because they consoli-
date the existing evidence on a topic. As a health or social care practitioner, you cannot be expected to read, evaluate, assimilate, and apply all

the information on any one topic even if you could find it in the first place! Since some literature reviews will be of a better quality than others, it is important that you check the way in which the review has been written so that you can ensure that a comprehensive approach has been undertaken.

Primary/empirical research

Primary/empirical research relates to individual studies that are undertaken in a planned and methodological way and for which **raw data** are collected. Patients or clients are often invited to participate in research studies in order to further knowledge and understanding of practice. There are generally considered to be two main types: quantitative and qualitative. These will now be discussed in detail.

Quantitative research

Quantitative research is a type of primary research sometimes called positivist research. It normally refers to studies that use methods of data collection that measure outcomes using numbers combined with statistical analysis.

 Quantitative research seeks to quantify or measure the items under exploration in the study.

You will come across quantitative research when you are looking for research about topics that can be **measured numerically**, for example, how many people quit smoking after a campaign, or how satisfied people are with some aspect of service provision. 'Tick boxes' and measurement scales are often used for this type of research.

Key features of quantitative research studies

- They tend to involve large numbers of participants.
- They are undertaken only when data can be measured or collected numerically.
- They often resemble a 'traditional experiment' or study – there is minimal or no involvement between the researcher and participant (the aim is to be objective).

- Other factors that could influence the results are kept to a minimum (called **confounding variables**).
- Data are analysed using statistical tests.
- The aim of quantitative research is to generalize findings to other contexts.

Sample size

Sample size in quantitative research tends to be large. *This is because, if the sample size is large, any significant findings are more likely to reflect what would occur in an average population.*

For example, you are likely to have greater confidence in a study comparing two treatment options in which many thousands of people had participated than a study conducted with just twenty participants.

Think about the last piece of research you read about. Consider how appropriate the sample size involved in the research was.

If the condition under investigation is unusual, sample size will inevitably be smaller. Paradoxically, however, you need to have a large sample size to be able to find out about the **incidence rate**.

Quantitative studies often use the terms 'random sampling' and/or 'random allocation'/'randomization' – these terms are often confused and it is important to recognize the difference between them.

Random sampling applies when all the members of a population have an equal chance of being selected. This ensures that the sample is not biased (there is no selection bias). Compare this with **convenience sampling,** which as its name suggests is where the sample is recruited from participants who are local or otherwise 'convenient' to the study.

Example from practice

A random sample of university students could be drawn from the university admission lists rather than from those attending lectures, given that all students will be on the admission list but not all will attend lectures. Any sample drawn from those who attend lectures will be biased rather than random. It is important to note that obtaining an unbiased sample in any research study is very difficult. A questionnaire might be sent to a random sample of the population, but unless there is a 100% **response rate**, the responses obtained will be biased (**non-responder bias**).

 Randomization/random allocation is used within a randomized controlled trial when participants in the study are not selected from the population at random but are allocated at random to one group within the study.

Randomization or random allocation

The process of allocating individuals at random (by chance) to groups, usually in a randomized controlled trial, to ensure that two or more groups in a trial are equal in terms of participant characteristics. We discuss this in more detail later in the chapter.

Experimental and non-experimental quantitative research

 Quantitative research can be divided into experimental and non-experimental research.

Experimental methods can be used to measure the effectiveness or action of an intervention (for example, smoking cessation interventions). In this case, quantitative methods could be used to compare how many people quit smoking in the intervention group and in the non-intervention group. This would be measured numerically, in months and years. The important thing here is that the experimenter controls who is allocated to which intervention. Hence we call it an experiment. **Non-experimental** research designs include questionnaires/surveys, for which participants respond to questions. Their responses can then be counted numerically – for example, 30% of those who responded to the survey had done X.

In principle, quantitative research is generally undertaken when you are looking to measure something and that something is suitable for numerical measurement. Let's look in more detail at some of the quantitative research designs that you are likely to encounter.

Types of experimental quantitative studies

Let's look at the experimental quantitative studies you may come across, starting with the randomized controlled trial (RCT). It is an important design and once you have understood the basic principles of an RCT, you will see more clearly how the other quantitative studies work.

Randomized controlled trials

> **Randomized controlled trials** *are a form of clinical trial, or scientific procedure, used to determine the effectiveness of a treatment, intervention or medicine. Participants who have the same condition or problem and who agree to enter the study are randomly allocated to two or more groups. Participants in each group receive either an intervention or no intervention. Any changes to their condition can be attributed to the intervention because of the otherwise equal nature of the groups.*

Randomized controlled trials are useful when you wish to determine whether a treatment or intervention is effective or better than an alternative intervention. In this case, you should search for RCTs in the first instance. If you find some RCTs, then you probably have good evidence about the effectiveness of your treatment or intervention. If you are unable to find any RCTs or a review of RCTs, you will not be able to discern whether the intervention or therapy works or not.

Key features of randomized controlled trials

- It is widely considered to be the most thorough ('gold standard') form of evidence when we are considering whether a treatment or intervention is effective.
- Participants are allocated by random allocation/randomization into two or more groups. This keeps differences to the groups to a minimum.
- An intervention is then given to one of the groups and not given to the other (control) group; the outcome of the two groups is then compared.

- If it is not possible to randomize participants in a research study and expose one group to a particular intervention (for example, for ethical reasons), then it is not possible to carry out an RCT.
- The sample sizes should be large enough to exclude the result being due just to chance.

Example from practice

The practice of swaddling babies used to be very common in many cultures and is still adhered to today in very cold climates. This practice was (and is) necessary to protect babies from the severe cold and as a means of keeping them safe when travelling. However, as different options have become available for protecting children, the question of whether the practice of swaddling is harmful to babies has become significant. For this reason, a team of researchers (Manaseki-Holland et al. 2010) undertook an RCT to determine whether swaddling babies has any negative effect on their growth and development. The researchers described the trial as follows:

> 1279 healthy new-borns in Ulaanbaatar, Mongolia, were allocated at birth to traditional swaddling or non-swaddling. The families received 7 months of home visits to collect data and monitor compliance. At 11 to 17 months of age, [the trial] was administered to 1100 children.
>
> (Manaseki-Holland et al. 2010: e1485)

Randomized controlled trials are generally considered to be the best way (and many people would say the only way) to determine whether a new treatment or intervention is effective or an established treatment is harmful or not. In the example above, the intervention investigated was the introduction of clothing and the control group was the standard practice of swaddling newborn babies.

The importance of random allocation/randomization

Participants are allocated into the different treatment groups of the trial at **random**. This is similar to tossing a coin. This ensures that participants are allocated into the different groups by chance rather than based on the preferences of the patients/clients or researchers. It is very important that neither the participants nor the researchers have any control or choice over the group to which participants are allocated. Today, this is generally done by computer.

Example continued . . .

If we take the Mongolian study, the process of randomization required that mothers of the babies did not have any input into which group their babies were entered into. One group was allocated to the traditional practice of swaddling while the second group was given extra warm layers of clothing. It must have been quite daunting for the mothers of the babies in the intervention group who were not swaddled but were dressed in extra layers of clothing, to go against years of traditional practice! When they agreed to participate in the study, they were informed that their baby could be allocated to either of the two groups.

Random allocation/randomization is important because the researcher is looking for differences between the treatment group and the control group as a result of the treatment or intervention. If the groups are randomly and equally allocated, then any differences in outcome can be said to be due to the intervention alone. This can only be determined if the different groups, which are commonly referred to as 'arms', of the trial are equal in all respects (such as age/sex/severity of condition) except for the treatment or intervention being researched. With smaller samples, randomization is sometimes modified using a process called **stratification** to ensure that the groups are equal in respect of age/ sex/severity of condition, which we discuss below.

Example continued . . .

In the case of the Mongolian babies, researchers were interested in whether the practice of swaddling had any effect on the babies' development compared with babies who had not been swaddled. If the babies had been randomized into two groups, there should have been no other differences between the babies in the two groups.

Why can't participants choose which group they want to be entered into?

If the research participants were allowed to choose which group of the RCT they wanted to enter, it is likely one of the groups would be more popular than the other(s), although it's not always possible to say which. This would lead to the different groups in the trial not being equal.

Without equal groups, it would not be possible to determine whether the differences in outcomes observed between the different treatment or control groups of the trial were due to the intervention or whether they were due to the differences in the characteristics of the participants who had self-selected into one group or another.

How can the groups in an RCT have similar characteristics after randomization?

With large sample sizes, the randomization process normally results in the creation of groups containing participants with similar characteristics. If it is particularly important that participants with specific characteristics are equally represented in all groups (for example, participants in certain age groups or those who care for relatives might have different lifestyle habits from those without children and you might want an equal number of these participants in each group), then a further form of randomization can be used. This is an additional statistical process that assists in ensuring that the groups are equal in respect of certain predefined criteria (for example, age, sex, ethnic group) that are relevant to the research, and this is called **stratification**, **matching** or **minimization**.

 Can you explain the difference between random sampling and randomization/ random allocation?

How does an RCT work?

Once participants in a trial have been randomly allocated and the groups are considered to be equal, the intervention, treatment or therapy is given to one group (the **intervention** group). This is often called the **independent variable**. A second group (sometimes called the non-intervention group) receives either the standard treatment or no treatment (the placebo – see below). The groups are then monitored and the differences between the groups noted. Given that the two groups of participants were randomly allocated and hence can be considered to be 'equal', any difference between the groups can be attributed to the effect of the intervention. The outcome measured is often called the **dependent variable**.

The **non-intervention** group may be:

- **A control group** who receive the established standard/normal treatment or intervention

- **A placebo group** who receive a dummy or sham drug or treatment, but the important thing is that the participants do not know this! If at all possible, neither the researcher running the trial nor the participants know which group they have been allocated to. Including a placebo group is, however, only **ethical** if non-treatment is not thought to be harmful to participants – let's say if there was genuine uncertainty as to the effectiveness of a treatment. This is called **blinding**.

*Blinding in a study can either be **double blind** – when neither the researcher nor participants know which group the participants are in, or **single blind** – when only the researchers know which group the participants are allocated to.*

This obviously depends on what the study is looking for and whether it is possible to blind either the researchers/data analysts or participants.

> **Example continued . . .**
>
> In the Mongolian study, there was a control group, a group of babies who received the traditional practice of swaddling. The intervention group was given extra layers of clothing. At the end of the trial, researchers looked to see what the differences in outcome were between the different groups in the trial – for example, what was the difference in growth and development between the babies who had been swaddled and those who had not? Because the groups were otherwise equal, we can say that any differences in outcome are likely to be attributable to the intervention versus control (clothing versus swaddling).

What is a null hypothesis and why do we have one?

A **null hypothesis** is usually stated when an RCT is designed. The null hypothesis is a starting point – it is a 'negatively' phrased statement that asserts that *there is no difference between the two groups*. The aim of the RCT is to determine whether this assertion (i.e. the null hypothesis) can be confirmed or rejected. If the results show that there is a difference between the control group and the intervention group, then the null hypothesis can be rejected.

Example continued . . .

In the Mongolian study, the researchers described the null hypothesis as follows:

The null hypothesis was that Mongolian infants not swaddled or swaddled tightly in a traditional setting (to >7 months of age) do not have significantly different scores for the Bayley Scales of Infant Development, Second Edition (BSID-II).

(Manaseki-Holland et al. 2010: e1485)

A flow diagram of the process of conducting an RCT for the Mongolian study babies is presented below:

Newborn babies were recruited in a clinic in Ulaanbaatar, Mongolia

Mothers of the babies who agreed to participate in the study were informed about the process of randomization. This population was then randomly allocated into two groups:

1. Group 1 babies carry on normal swaddling practice
2. Group 2 babies receive additional clothing but are not swaddled

The rate and range of movement and overall development of the babies in the different groups are then compared at set points in the study. Any differences in outcomes are attributed to swaddling or non-swaddling, given that the groups were randomized and therefore otherwise equal

In the Mongolian study, the researchers found that there were no differences in the growth and development of the babies in the two groups. They described their results as follows. (Note the term 'significant' is a statistical term that we discuss later in this chapter.)

No significant between-group differences were found in mean scaled mental and psychomotor developmental scores.

(Manaseki-Holland et al. 2010: e1485)

The Mongolian swaddling study illustrates how an RCT can be used to determine whether an intervention is beneficial, harmful or indeed makes no difference.

Differences between the two or more groups in an RCT are often expressed as a **risk ratio** or **odds ratio**. To understand these terms, consider a study that explored the effect of a new intervention to help people quit smoking. In the intervention group, 40 out of 100 people stop smoking. In the control group, only 20 out of 100 people stop smoking. To calculate how much more likely you are to stop smoking if you take the new intervention, we take the proportion of people who stop with the new drug (40/100) and divide by the proportion of people in the control group who stop (20/100). The answer is 2, so we can say that people are twice as likely to stop smoking if they use the intervention. This figure is the risk ratio. The odds ratio is slightly less intuitive and is not often used for reporting trials and is defined in the glossary. Randomized controlled trials can only be used when it is possible to allocate participants within a group at random and administer a treatment or intervention to one group and not to the other. When this cannot be done, often for ethical reasons, a modified experiment may be considered.

Quasi-experiments

Quasi-experiments have some of the features of an RCT but not all of them. They are usually carried out when it is not possible to undertake an RCT.

Example from practice

If you were exploring infant nutrition, it would not be acceptable or ethical to ask one group of mothers to abstain from breastfeeding their babies in order to make a comparison with another group of mothers who were asked to breastfeed.

Quasi-experiments are most useful *when you need to determine cause and effect, but are not able to undertake a randomized controlled trial.*

The important point about quasi-experiments is that they share many of the same characteristics as an RCT. They deviate from this design usually when circumstances demand that adherence to the RCT method is not practical or ethical.

Example from practice

Say you want to find out whether a new style of parenting class is effective. Because of the nature of childcare, it is not possible to undertake an RCT. Instead, you implement the new style of class with one group of parents who have enrolled on a parenting class and compare the results with another group in another area who have not completed this class. You can see that the two groups in the experiment are not equal – the parents in one class might come from different sociological groups than those in another and while you might allow for this by selecting similar areas in which to conduct the study, you will not achieve equal groups as you would in an RCT. Therefore, if the outcomes for the parents who experienced the new style of parenting class were different from the outcomes of those who did not, you would not be able to determine whether the differences were due to other factors.

In a quasi-experiment, therefore, it is not possible to say with as much certainty that the outcome was due to the intervention administered. While non-randomized experiments will provide you with evidence, this is generally thought to be **second-best evidence** if you are looking to determine the effectiveness of an intervention.

Non-experimental quantitative methods

Cohort studies and **case control studies** try to link up the causes of diseases and/or interventions and/or social situations. Cohort studies and case control studies were first used to observe the effects of an exposure (e.g. smoking) on the health of those observed.

Cohort and case control studies are most useful when you need information about the likely causes of a disease or other problems but you are unable to perform an experiment. For example, you wish to determine whether excessive alcohol leads to dementia. You cannot, of course, perform an experiment to find this out but you can follow up those who do drink and compare the rate of dementia with those who do not.

Key features of cohort and case control studies

- They are used most often to find the causes or impact of disease.
- They are then followed up in order to observe the effect of the exposure to, for example, smoking nicotine on the health and social wellbeing of those observed.

Cohort studies are observational studies. These studies attempt to discover the causes or risk factors of a disease or problem when it is not possible to carry out an experiment.

A cohort study involves a **group of people who have all been exposed to a particular event, risk or lifestyle** (for example, they all smoke or have a particular disability). Individuals in the cohort who smoke and who develop lung cancer, say, are then compared with those who don't smoke. The cohort study compares the incidence in both groups and draws conclusions about the association of the risk, event or lifestyle factor. However, because the groups were not formed by random allocation, any observed differences between the two groups at the end of the study period are not as easily attributable to the exposure as if the study had been an RCT.

Example 1: In a cohort study, Teng et al. (2017) followed up a very large cohort (54 'million person years' between 1981 and 2011) and were able to identify patterns in cancer incidence and type by socio-economic group. They identified the contribution of cancer to the mortality gap between high and low socio-economic groups in high-income countries.

Example 2: In another well-known cohort study, Allen et al. (2009) identified that women who drink even modest amounts of alcohol are more at risk of developing breast cancer than their non-drinking counterparts. Women attending a clinic for breast cancer screening were followed up and the drinking habits of those who went on to develop breast cancer were compared with those who did not develop the disease.

The Million Women Study has been described previously. In 1996–2001 a total of 1.3 million middle-aged women who attended breast cancer screening clinics in the United Kingdom completed a questionnaire that asked for socio-demographic and other personal information, including how much wine, beer, and spirits they drank on average each week. Information on whether the wine consumed was red, white or both was also recorded. In a follow-up survey, done about 3 years after recruitment, study participants were again asked to report the usual number of alcoholic drinks consumed per week.

(Allen et al. 2009: 296–297)

This cohort study demonstrated that there was a strong association between alcohol consumption and the development of breast cancer.

The following is a flow diagram of the process of conducting a cohort study:

Cohort of people who all experienced the same exposure/experience

This cohort is followed up to observe the effect of this exposure

The cohort may be compared with the control group who did not experience this exposure.

A **case control study** works the other way round to a cohort study. People (cases) who have a condition are studied and compared with cases that do not. You might, for example, explore the alcohol consumption of women who have developed breast cancer and compare it to the consumption of women who do not have the disease.

In a case control study, patients/clients with a particular condition are studied *and* compared with *others who do not have that condition in an effort to establish whether a particular exposure is responsible for the condition.*

In a case control study, the **researchers identify those who have developed the disease (the cases)** and compare them with those who did not (control). If the cases have had greater exposure to a particular factor compared with the control group, it suggests an association between that factor and the disease.

Example

In 1954, Doll and Hill carried out a case control study of lung cancer. In their study, patients/clients were traced back to see what could have caused the disease. They designed a questionnaire that was administered to patients/clients with suspected lung, liver or bowel cancer. Those administering the questionnaire were not aware which of the diseases was suspected in which patients/clients. It became clear from the questionnaires that those who were later confirmed to have lung cancer were also confirmed smokers. Those who did not have lung cancer did not smoke. Clearly, it would not have been ethical to undertake an RCT to explore the causes of lung cancer, as it would not have been possible to randomize a group of non-smokers and ask one group to start smoking!

The following is a flow diagram of the process of conducting a case control study:

Individuals with a specific condition or situation are identified

The circumstances that led up to the development/progress of this condition are then explored

Questionnaires/surveys/cross-sectional studies

Questionnaires and surveys are a popular type of (usually) quantitative research that you have probably come across yourself. They provide a snapshot of participants' responses to questions on a particular topic at a given point in time.

Questionnaires/surveys are studies in which a sample is taken at one point in time (cross-section of a population) from a defined group of people and observed/assessed.

Questionnaires/surveys are most useful when you are looking for evidence of the frequency of a particular activity, or information about a large group of people. Remember that questionnaires/survey studies have many limitations as outlined below, and the results of these should be viewed with caution.

Key features of questionnaires/surveys

- They can be used to collect data in RCTs, cohort and case control studies.
- If they are poorly designed, they will lead to misleading conclusions!
- They will only collect useful data if the questions have been well tested and piloted.
- They can be quantitative (numerical or rating scales), qualitative (free text boxes) or mixed.
- They can be administered by post, by email/electronic surveys or in person/interview.

Potential problems with questionnaires/surveys

- A long questionnaire might be discarded by participants before completing it in full.

- Respondents might misunderstand complicated or badly worded questions.
- Postal questionnaires have the additional disadvantage that there is likely to be a low response rate.
- If large sections of the target population do not respond, the overall quality of data collected will be poor.
- It is often not possible to access a fully representative sample for the distribution of a questionnaire.
- The completed questionnaires will contain information from a selection of, but not a random sample of, participants and will therefore not provide a complete picture of the target population.

Example 1: If you identified that illicit drugs users also experience high levels of anxiety, it would be tempting to conclude that use of illicit drugs increases anxiety. However, perhaps the reverse is true and those with high levels of anxiety resort to illicit drug use.

Example 2: if you distribute the questionnaire in a shopping centre on a Saturday, you will reach a different population than if the questionnaire is distributed on a weekday. Similarly, you will likely get a different group of people depending on the time at which the questionnaire is distributed. Distributing the questionnaire on different days of the week at different times would help to overcome this.

Example 3: If you distribute a questionnaire via text, social media or email, a different population might respond than if you posted it.

Data analysis in quantitative research

 There are two main types of statistics: descriptive *and* inferential.

Descriptive statistics describe the data given in the paper. These statistics should clearly describe the main results, such as how many people answered 'yes' to a particular question or what the most common response to a question was.

The results will typically be reported as follows:

- **Mean:** this is the average when all the results are added up and divided by the number of participants. **Example:** if the results for five participants are 25, 35, 20, 20, 40, then the average score will be the total of these (140) divided by the number of participants (5), giving a mean score of 28.

- **Median:** the middle value if the results are ranked from lowest to highest. **Example:** of the following 11 results, 1, 1, 2, 3, 3, **4**, 5, 6, 6, 7, 7, the number 4 is in the middle and is the median.
- **Mode:** this is the number that occurs most often. Example: of the following 10 results, 1, 1, 2, **3, 3, 3,** 6, 7, 8, 8, the number 3 is the mode as it occurs three times.
- **Percentages** are also used. This indicates how many out of 100, such that 65 out of 100 = 65%.
- **Standard deviation:** this shows how spread out the data is from the average (mean). The further the data is spread out, the higher the standard deviation. If the deviation is small, then most results are close to the average (mean). This is often represented in a distribution curve.

In contrast, **inferential statistics** generalize to the wider population. In other words, they determine the extent to which the results obtained from the sample in the research have any relevance to the **wider population** as a whole.

- Inferential statistics do more than describe a sample, they infer or predict how likely that is to apply to the wider population.
- The larger the sample, the more sure you can be that the sample prevalence is close to the population prevalence.

Example

At the time of an election, opinion polls are used to predict the overall result of the election. These polls are based on a small sample of voters but are used with varying effect to predict the overall result.

Confidence intervals

You might see two numbers written besides the main findings or results in brackets. These are called confidence intervals.

Say you want to know how many people are going to vote for the Green Party. If you asked 10 people and two people told you they were going to vote for this party, you would be fairly uncertain about how the voting was likely to go; however, if you asked 100 people and 20 people told you they were going to vote for the Green Party, you would have more of an idea. If you asked 1000 people and 200 were going to vote for the Green

Party, you would have a more precise prediction still. In each case, you are using a sample of the electorate to predict how the whole electorate or population is going to vote. In research, we take a sample to make generalizations about the population as a whole.

Confidence intervals express the uncertainty of our estimate. They use the results of a study to make a prediction about what the 'true' result in the whole population might be.

Confidence intervals are usually (but arbitrarily) 95% confidence intervals. A reasonable, though strictly incorrect interpretation is that the 95% confidence interval gives the range in which the population effect lies. A wide confidence interval implies a lack of certainty or precision about the true population effect and is commonly found in studies with few participants. You will see confidence intervals expressed as an estimate after the result found in a study (for example, 6% of students responded positively to an item in a questionnaire CI 5–7%).

Thinking of the samples above, the first sample of 10 people would have more uncertainty than the third example in which 1000 people were consulted. This is expressed as a confidence interval, which quantifies the uncertainty. So, if two people out of 10 told you they were going to vote for the Green Party, the confidence intervals would likely be wide. The best estimate would be that 20% of the population would vote for the Green Party but you would not be very certain about this and would express that uncertainty by giving a range of percentages of people who might vote Green – for example, 4–56%. This means that we can be 95% sure that somewhere between 4% and 56% of the population will vote for the Green Party. In the sample where 1000 people were consulted, again the best estimate would be that 20% would vote for the Green Party but because the sample is larger, the confidence intervals would be smaller – for example, 18–23%. This means that we can be 95% certain that somewhere between 18% and 23% of the population will vote Green. Confidence intervals are worked out using a statistical formula and are calculated with a 95% confidence interval. This means that we can be 95% sure that the confidence intervals are between the ranges stated.

- The smaller the interval or range, the more confident you can be that the results in the study reflect the result you would find in the larger population.

- By using a formula, the upper and lower confidence intervals can be calculated. A **95% confidence interval** means that we can be 95% sure that the true population prevalence lies between the lower and upper confidence intervals.

Probability value (*p*-value)

Statistics are often described using the ***p-value*** or probability. It is related to the **statistical significance** of results or findings.

The p-value expresses the probability of the difference shown between the groups in an experiment being due to chance. It is important to determine the likelihood that the findings are down to chance in any research.

The lower the *p*-value, the less likely it is that a finding is due to chance. If the *p*-value is less than 0.05 (1:20), we say the finding is unlikely to be due to chance. If the *p*-value is much less than 0.05 (1:20), say, $p = 0.005$ (1:200), then the finding is even more unlikely to be due to chance.

Example

You undertake an RCT to compare different ways of helping people quit smoking. Normally in an RCT, you would give an intervention to one group and not to the other and then examine the differences in outcome between the groups.

However, if both groups are treated with the standard treatment, you will likely see a variety of outcomes in each group due to natural differences between the groups. Thus, you administer an intervention to one of the groups and observe the different outcomes of the two groups. The *p*-value can then be calculated to determine whether the differences in outcome observed are due to chance or not.

To calculate the *p*-value, we refer to the **null hypothesis**. In the philosophy of science, we can never prove something is true, only disprove something. For this reason, we develop a hypothesis that is the opposite of what we actually believe – this is the null hypothesis. This is a phrase that is used when you state (in order to test it) that there is no relationship between the different elements (or **variables**) under study. For example, *'there is no difference in outcomes for parents who attend parenting classes and those who do not'*. This hypothesis can be tested using the results from the study when the different groups are compared and calculated using a statistical test, such as the chi-squared test (χ^2-test). A p-value of 0.05, for example, means there is a 1 in 20 chance of seeing these results if the null hypothesis were true. So, this means that there is a relationship between the variables. It is important to remember that this does not indicate a causal relationship, i.e. that one variable caused the other, but just that the two occur together.

This basic outline of some of the statistics you might use is intended to help you understand how they are used and tell us about the strength or not of a set of results. They help us to understand if a particular piece of research helps us to answer a question. Next time you read a paper containing statistics, ask yourself what the statistics say about the results and the strength of evidence presented.

Qualitative studies

Qualitative studies typically **do not seek to quantify or measure** the items under exploration using numbers as in quantitative research. Instead, they aim to **explore an issue in depth**. They are often carried out on an area or topic where little research evidence exists.

The aim of all qualitative approaches is to explore the meaning of and develop in-depth understanding of the research topic as experienced by the participants in the research.

The results of qualitative research are not expressed in percentages and numbers but as **words** in the form of **descriptive themes.**

Qualitative research is most useful when you are looking for in-depth insight or answers to questions that cannot be answered numerically, when you want to ask why?, how? or what?

Think of an issue in your own practice for which you could explore a qualitative question relating to the experience, perception or understanding of that issue.

Key qualities of qualitative studies

- These types of studies are sometimes referred to as naturalistic research.
- Researchers seek to understand the *whole* of an experience and gain insight into that experience.
- The data collected is not numerical but is collected, often through interview, using the words and descriptions of the participants.
- There is no use of statistics in qualitative research; the results are **descriptive** and **interpretative**.
- They do not set out to look for specific ideas, hoping to confirm pre-existing beliefs. Instead, they code the data and build themes according to ideas arising from within it. This process is often referred to as being **inductive**.
- The generation of themes, although rigorous, is **interpretative and subjective**, depending on the insight of the researcher.
- The researcher cannot achieve complete objectivity because he or she is the data collection tool (for example, the interviewer) and subjectively interprets the data collected. This is acknowledged in the research process and steps are taken to maintain **credibility** and **trustworthiness** in this process as far as possible.
- Sample sizes tend to be small. A small sample is required because in-depth understanding (rather than statistical analysis) is sought from information-rich participants.
- **Participants recruited** to a qualitative study tend not to be selected at random, but instead are selected because they have had exposure to or experience of the phenomenon of interest in that particular study.

This type of sampling is referred to as **purposive sampling** and this leads to the selection of information-rich participants who can contribute to answering the research question. Other approaches to sampling in qualitative research are **convenience sampling** – made up of people who are easily accessible; **theoretical sampling** – where the sample (used in grounded theory) is determined according to the needs of the study; and **snowball sampling** – where the sample is developed as new potential participants are identified as the study progresses. For example, contacts of participants already involved in the research may be invited to enter the study if they have the relevant experience.

Large numbers of participants are rarely recruited (and are not necessarily appropriate) in qualitative research.

The richness of qualitative data arises from **the dialogue between the researcher and the participant** and the insights obtained through this process are only possible because of the **interaction** between the two. For example, the interviewer may probe the interviewee about his or her responses to a question and phrase the next question as a direct response to the reply received. **Subjectivity is required** for the researcher to gain an insight into the topic under investigation – objectivity is not the aim.

Qualitative data analysis is **open to interpretation**. Because the researcher is involved in, and indeed shapes, both the data collection and analysis process, it is not possible for the researcher to remain detached from the data collected. The concept of **reflexivity** is important and refers to the acknowledgement by the qualitative researcher that this process of enquiry is necessarily open to interpretation and that **detachment** from the focus of the research is **neither desirable nor possible**.

Examples of qualitative research questions

- What it is like for a patient/client who has had a stroke?
- What is the lived experience of mothers forced to leave their home due to repossession?
- What is the experience of physiotherapy students on placement in the community?

 See if you can find a qualitative study that relates to your own professional practice or specialism. You may find it useful to use the search terms 'experiences' or 'perceptions' of your patients/clients or families.

Different approaches to qualitative research

The most commonly used **data collection methods** in qualitative research are:

- In-depth interviews
- Focus groups
- Questionnaires using open-ended questions.

There are a wide variety of approaches to qualitative research. You are likely to encounter many different approaches when you read the literature. Some are simply described in the literature as 'qualitative studies', while others are named according to the particular qualitative approach that is followed. These are outlined below. It is useful to recognize these different approaches and to understand why one approach was selected for a specific research question.

Grounded theory

Grounded theory is a way of finding out about what happens in a social setting and then making wider generalizations about the way things happen. The purpose of grounded theory is to generate a theory from the data and observations that are made. It is a 'bottom-up' or inductive approach in which data is collected and analysed and then used to help explain why things happen in social life. **Grounded theory is most useful** when you want to explore an area that has not been studied extensively and you are looking to develop theory about what is happening in a particular context.

Example

Giles et al. (2016) undertook a grounded theory study in order to explore (and develop a theory about) the factors that influence decision-making when family members are present during resuscitation. The researchers conducted interviews with healthcare professionals, relatives and, where appropriate, the patient. The researchers found that the values and preferences of staff influenced the involvement of relatives and hence involvement in decision-making varied greatly.

Phenomenology

Phenomenology is the study of the 'lived experience' or what it is actually like to live with a particular condition or experience. Such studies often use in-depth interviews as the means of data collection, as they allow the participant the opportunity to explore and describe their experience within an interview setting. **Phenomenology is most useful** when you want to find out about individual experiences of an illness, social situation, concept or event.

Example

Maltby et al. (2016) undertook a phenomenological study in which they explored the experiences of students from low- and high-income countries of a nursing exchange. They interviewed 44 students about their experiences and from the analysis of these interviews were able to identify common themes. They found an increase in cultural competence among those who had participated in the exchange and advocated exploring ways of increasing understanding of diversity within the curriculum for those unable to travel and study abroad.

Ethnography

Ethnography is the study of human culture. An ethnographic study focuses on a community (i.e. a specific group of people) in order to gain insight into how its members behave. Observation or participant observation and/or in-depth interviews may be undertaken to achieve this. As it seeks to observe phenomena as they occur in real time, a true ethnographic study is a time-consuming process. **Ethnography is most useful** when you want to find out about a culture or way of life of a group of people in order to understand why they act and behave in the way they do.

Example

Sullivan et al. (2016) conducted an ethnographical study in which they explored how women in Ghana perceive the support they receive when they have an obstetric fistula. The researchers undertook observations and interviews with women affected by obstetric fistulas, their partners, and healthcare professionals. By observing and finding out about the everyday life of the women and their professional and informal carers, they observed that many women found travelling to receive medical attention both difficult and costly. On arrival there was often no sustenance and treatment practices were variable.

Action research

Action research is the process by which practitioners or researchers work together to address issues that arise in everyday practice in order to develop a systematic approach to implementing and evaluating change. Action research is a cyclical method of planning, implementing, and evaluating change and development in the working environment. Action research is often designed and conducted by practitioners who wish to to improve their own practice. **Action research is useful when** you need to generate improvements in organizations that are not in the form of research findings, but are generated as solutions from within.

Example

Bulman et al. (2016) undertook an action research study to explore the use of reflection among nurse educators. They confirmed the usefulness of a flexible toolbox of resources for reflection in practice and the need for opportunities to share concerns and a facilitative approach through which these concerns could be addressed.

Discourse analysis

You may also come across **discourse analysis,** an approach that analyses the use of language in order to understand meaning in complex areas. **Discourse analysis is most useful when** the researcher wants to gain understanding of complex phenomena. Using analysis of the language people use in day-to-day communication helps to determine the reality of their beliefs and values rather than what they might say when questioned or asked for their opinions.

Example

Caddick et al. (2017) carried out a discourse analysis of how lorry drivers understand their health needs. This study involved analysis of conversations, often undertaken in the cab of the lorry while on the road.

Concept analysis

Concept analysis is used to explore concepts that are often interpreted differently within practice and the literature. A specific framework is often used to guide a concept analysis. The antecedents (what comes before), attributes, consequences, interrelationships, and referents (what the word stands for) of each concept are determined. In addition, similarities and differences are usually identified and then a definition is given.

Example

Castro et al. (2016) carried out a concept analysis into patient empowerment, patient participation, and patient-centredness in hospital care.

After reading this section, try to summarize your learning on literature reviews, quantitative and qualitative research methodologies. If you are unclear, read the section again or discuss it with a colleague or fellow student.

Which type of research is best?

There has been much debate in the research literature on the merits of the different approaches to research (i.e. quantitative or qualitative), with some researchers claiming that one is better than the other. In this book, we argue that this debate is meaningless because quantitative and qualitative approaches look at different things, or different aspects of the same problem – it is not possible or helpful to say that one is better than the other. In addition, many researchers use mixed methods to approach a research question, thus enabling the question to be explored from different perspectives. This increases the potential for the research to be more acceptable and relevant to practice.

There are many similarities between quantitative and qualitative approaches to research. Both start with a research question and select the appropriate methodology to answer that question. In all research papers, the methods used to undertake the research should be clearly explained and the results clearly presented. This **research process** is described earlier and is the same process used to describe a systematic review or a primary research paper.

The various research methods are outlined above in order to illustrate that it is not possible to use qualitative methods to address a question where quantitative methods are more appropriate and vice versa. Different problems require different types of research. It is important that as users of research, we find the most appropriate type of research to suit our needs in a particular context.

It is most important that the most appropriate research methodology is used to address what you wish to research.

What does the term 'hierarchy of evidence' mean?

There is general agreement that a 'hierarchy of evidence' exists – that is, that **research can be ranked in order of importance** and that some forms of research evidence are stronger than others in addressing some types of research questions.

There are different hierarchies of evidence depending on what you need to find out.

However, as you can deduce from the previous discussion, there is **no one single hierarchy of evidence**.

The 'traditional' hierarchy of evidence for determining effective treatment puts systematic reviews and randomized controlled trials at the top and anecdotal opinion at the bottom, as shown here (Sackett et al. 1996).

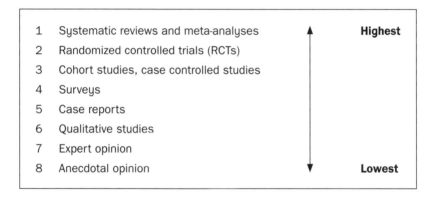

1	Systematic reviews and meta-analyses	▲	**Highest**
2	Randomized controlled trials (RCTs)		
3	Cohort studies, case controlled studies		
4	Surveys		
5	Case reports		
6	Qualitative studies		
7	Expert opinion		
8	Anecdotal opinion	▼	**Lowest**

To make sense of this hierarchy, we first need to acknowledge that (systematic) **literature reviews almost always provide the strongest evidence**. Therefore, most people would agree that a review should always be at the top of any hierarchy. So *position 1* in the hierarchy is not really up for debate. However, if we go to *position 2*, the second ranked item is the RCT, and this is where it gets more interesting. In the hierarchy of evidence above, the RCT is the next best form of evidence in the absence of a (systematic) literature review. This might be the case **if** the research question you are interested in can be answered using an RCT, for example, if you need to find out about the effectiveness of one intervention or treatment over another. Moving down to *positions 3–8*, further different types of evidence are given, with qualitative studies and expert opinion very low down the ranking.

Can you identify any limitation of this type of hierarchy?

The limitation of this type of hierarchy is that it is **only** relevant if you are looking for evidence to determine whether a treatment or intervention is effective or not and therefore answerable using an RCT or review of RCTs as the best available evidence. We have seen earlier in this chapter how many research questions are not best addressed using RCTs or even quantitative studies at all. For those questions that cannot be answered by an RCT, this hierarchy is clearly not appropriate. It can therefore be misleading to consider just one hierarchy of evidence. In fact, what we really need are several hierarchies, which suit the different research questions we are likely to come across. In relation to public health and social policy, Parkhurst and Abeysinghe (2016) recommend that rather than adhering to a single hierarchy of evidence to judge what constitutes 'good' evidence for policy, it is more useful to consider evidence in relation to appropriateness.

Determining which evidence is best for your research question

We have emphasized throughout this book that it is important you to work out what type of information you require and that you should seek to find this information in the first instance. If you wish to determine the benefits or not of a particular practice, then the 'traditional' hierarchy of evidence will work and you will be looking for RCTs (after reviews of RCTs) in the first instance. If your question is not about whether an intervention or therapy works or not, then you need to think more broadly about the type of evidence you need. Elsewhere, Aveyard (2010) refers to **developing your own 'hierarchy of evidence'** to address the particular research question you are interested in. Noyes (2010) argues from a similar position and points out that different forms of evidence are valuable in different contexts. In some contexts, qualitative research will be more useful than quantitative research – for example, if you want to find out about patient or client experience so that a service can be improved. In these cases, qualitative research would be in *position 2* rather than *position 6* and the RCT would be ranked lower down, if it appeared at all!

Noyes (2010: 530) gives an example of a hierarchy of evidence that could help us understand client or patient experience. The hierarchy of **'views and experiences of interventions and services'** is given below:

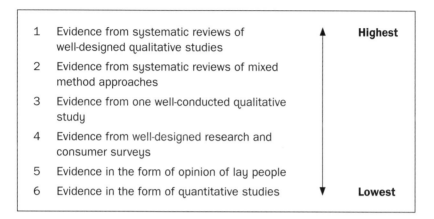

1   Evidence from systematic reviews of well-designed qualitative studies | **Highest**

2   Evidence from systematic reviews of mixed method approaches

3   Evidence from one well-conducted qualitative study

4   Evidence from well-designed research and consumer surveys

5   Evidence in the form of opinion of lay people

6   Evidence in the form of quantitative studies | **Lowest**

Noyes' (2010) hierarchy works well for research questions that are looking at qualitative experiences researched using qualitative methods and might be useful for the following question: *What is it like to enter the UK as a migrant worker?* If you want to find out what it is like to enter the UK as a migrant worker, you would need to find evidence of the experience of those workers. Therefore, qualitative studies, probably using a phenomenological approach, would be at the top of your hierarchy of evidence.

However, there are other research questions for which neither the 'traditional' or the 'views and experiences' hierarchy would be helpful. For example, let's say you are a public health specialist and need to find out whether people who have taken a particular drug are more at risk of a particular condition. Let's take, for example, thalidomide, which was prescribed in the 1960s to pregnant women as an anti-sickness medication and which was found to lead to malformations in the babies of women who took the drug. In this case, an RCT would not be appropriate as it would not be ethical to randomly allocate participants to receive either thalidomide or a placebo once you already had your suspicions about thalidomide. Instead, you would need to look for other types of quantitative studies – case controlled trials or cohort studies that explore the effects of a particular exposure on the population in question. Thus cohort studies or case control studies would be at the top of your hierarchy in this instance.

The hierarchy of evidence (adapted from Noyes 2010) for **determining whether something works or not when it would be incorrect to undertake an RCT** is as follows:

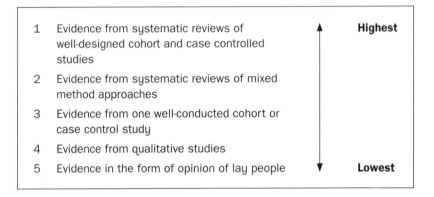

1 Evidence from systematic reviews of well-designed cohort and case controlled studies — Highest

2 Evidence from systematic reviews of mixed method approaches

3 Evidence from one well-conducted cohort or case control study

4 Evidence from qualitative studies

5 Evidence in the form of opinion of lay people — Lowest

Let's take another example. Imagine you want to find out whether public sector workers wash their hands prior to contact with their clients or patients. You would need to find evidence of what happens in practice through descriptions of care undertaken, or better still of observations of the care delivered. Therefore, studies of observation of or accounts of care delivery would be at the top of your hierarchy of evidence in this instance.

The hierarchy of evidence (adapted from Noyes 2010) for **determining whether public sector workers wash their hands** is as follows:

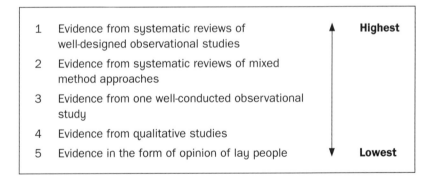

1 Evidence from systematic reviews of well-designed observational studies — Highest

2 Evidence from systematic reviews of mixed method approaches

3 Evidence from one well-conducted observational study

4 Evidence from qualitative studies

5 Evidence in the form of opinion of lay people — Lowest

As a final example in this section, say you want to determine how many students use illicit drugs while attending university. You would need to find questionnaires/surveys that have explored this aspect of student life.

While the data collected from questionnaires can be unreliable, in this instance there really is no other way to collect the data. Therefore, questionnaires/surveys would be at the top of your hierarchy of evidence.

The following is a hierarchy of evidence (adapted from Noyes 2010) for **identifying prevalence of drug use within a university population.**

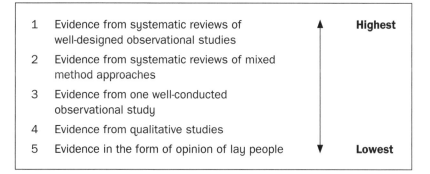

It should be clear from these examples that there is no one 'hierarchy of evidence' that works for all research questions. As suggested above, it is far better if you identify your 'own hierarchy of evidence' (Aveyard 2010), according to what evidence you need to address your own research question.

What about using secondary sources?

Secondary sources are those that report the findings of other people's work without giving full details of the work they discuss.

A secondary source is a source that does not report the data from a primary research study directly but it might refer to the study without giving full details or the authors may have paraphrased (put it into their own words). A secondary source is therefore a step removed from the ideas you are referring to.

Example

A report in the *British Medical Journal* (BMJ) might refer to a systematic review published by the Cochrane Collaboration. The BMJ report would

> be the secondary source and the Cochrane Collaboration report, the primary source. You may see it written as: 'Author A (2015) cited in Author B (2017)'.

- You are advised to access the primary source wherever possible and the use of **secondary sources should be avoided** wherever possible.
- If you rely on a secondary report and you do not access the original report, there is potential for you to miss any error in the way in which the initial source was reported and interpreted.
- Therefore, where you need to quote from another source, you are always advised to **access the original paper** rather than to refer to a report of it, unless it is not possible to get hold of the primary source, for example, if it is out of print or an unpublished doctoral thesis.

Let's say that the author (Author B) of a paper you are reading cites the work of a well-known author (Author A) who has done a lot of work in the area. If you refer to the work of Author A without accessing the original work, you are using a secondary source. You are relying on the interpretation of Author B to inform you about the work of Author A. You can see how this could lead to misinterpretation and this is why it should be avoided. Unless you read the original work by Author A, you are relying on Author B's interpretation of Author A's work.

Access the following example of the pitfalls of using secondary sources without accessing the primary source: Bradshaw and Price (2006).

We will not describe their work here (that would make us a secondary source). So we suggest you read it for yourselves.

Use of policy and guidelines

You are likely to come across a range of guidelines and policies in your practice. Ideally, these guidelines and policies are developed from the best available evidence. They should be written in a user-friendly way so that you can apply the evidence easily in your professional setting. They should have clearly stated authors, be dated, and have a review date.

See Chapter 7 and our useful websites section for more information about use of policy and guidelines.

There are often clinical and professional guidelines specific to individual professions, or even specific disorders.

Check your own organization's evidence-based policy or guidelines. It is also worth accessing those of other societies, colleges, and organizations specific to your profession or specialty.

You might also find that research evidence is integrated into other user-friendly publications. This means that you do not always have to locate the **'raw' data** from the research but instead search for publications that have cited evidence relevant to a particular context. Examples of such publications are:

- Government or professional organizations' policy, reports, guidance or standards
- NICE guidelines, which are frequently compiled with close reference to Cochrane and Campbell Collaboration reviews
- Care pathways or protocols
- Results from audits
- Reports from international, national or local organizations
- Information from trusted websites
- Blog shots (e.g. from Cochrane circulated on social media)
- Patient/client information leaflets.

As with other forms of evidence, it is important that these forms of evidence are evaluated – we explore this further in Chapter 6.

Non-research-based evidence

As stated previously, evidence will not always exist for your research question. This could be when you are unable to identify a focused question you can 'ask of the literature'. Or it could be that there is complexity, circumstances or context individual to the particular patient/client or situation, or you need to act in a novel situation. In such cases, you will have to use alternative forms of evidence (such as intuition, expert opinion, reflective judgement, discussion papers, and so on) to address the question you seek to answer at that moment. In this case, it is especially important that you assess the quality of the evidence that you have, as we will discuss in Chapter 6. When you use non-research evidence in your assignments (when that is all that is available) or practice (because of time or complexity issues), remember that it is not strong evidence *even if it is the best available*. It would be good practice if, at a later point, you looked for better quality direct or indirect research evidence that would better inform you if a similar situation were to arise again.

In summary

You will likely encounter a wide range of research evidence when you seek to address research questions that arise in your practice. It is important that you can recognize different types of research and understand when and why different approaches are used. There is no easy formula for determining what evidence is best in any given context – you need to consider carefully the types of evidence that will meet your needs. There is no one hierarchy of evidence; we suggest you develop your own in any given situation.

We will discuss how you search for and make sense of what you come across in the next two chapters. It is important that you are aware that different types of research evidence will assist you in addressing different types of questions that arise in practice.

Key points

1 You are likely to encounter a wide range of research and other information that is relevant to your specific question.
2 It is important that you can understand the key characteristics of a piece of research.
3 It is important to identify the types of research and other information that you need to address your question.
4 You may come across a wide range of evidence – it is important that you can recognize what you read and use it appropriately.
5 Traditional hierarchies of evidence only apply if you are looking for evidence of effectiveness.
6 Consider what the hierarchy of evidence is for your particular situation or context.
7 Other forms of information besides research are available, but you should ensure they are of the highest quality and – *where they can be* – are based on the best available evidence.

Quiz questions

1 What type of research study do you need to find if you are interested in whether a treatment or care intervention is effective?
2 What type of research study do you need to find if you are interested in patients' or clients' experiences?
3 What type of research study do you need to find if you are interested in possible causes of disease or illness?

5 How do I find relevant evidence to support my practice and learning?

In this chapter, we will consider:

- What evidence to look for – identifying your focus/keywords/search terms
- How to use the Internet, databases, and library
- How to search for literature
- How to increase, refine or reduce the results of a search
- How to use more advanced search techniques: hints and tips
- Using experts, specialists, and colleagues
- What to include and what to reject.

Where do I find relevant information? There are two things you need to do to find relevant information:

1 Focus the topic and refine the question
2 Search for evidence.

We look at each of these in turn.

Focusing the topic and refining the question

You may have a broad idea of the topic, relating to a decision you have made or need to make, but have yet to identify what exactly you need to focus on to answer your question. When you are looking for research to address a topic, a clear question will help you to decide if it is relevant and worth reading (Stern et al. 2014). You may have a more specific interest in mind that has arisen out of your academic studies, or an assignment you need to write, or an issue that has been raised in practice. We have already emphasized that the evidence you search for will depend on the question you need to answer. However, it is also important to focus what you need to find out so that you are not inundated with information.

Example

A broad topic may be suicide risk, but what exactly are you interested in? Is it risk factors in a particular group such as prisoners, or the experience of parents of teenagers who are at risk of suicide, or the prevalence of suicide risk in adults with chronic illness?

In Chapter 2, we discussed the information revolution and how as practitioners we are inundated with information about our practice. As can be seen above, if you undertake searches on 'broad' topics such as suicide, diabetes or child protection, you will get a very high number of results (hits) from your search and the results might be unmanageable. You have probably found this already when using search engines such as Google. If you ask for information on a particular country or event, you may get thousands of hits. When you refine this to something more specific, you will come closer to finding what you are looking for. It is the same within health and social care.

Consider what area of practice you are exploring. Your enquiry may relate to: assessment, screening, diagnosis, prognosis, prevention, interventions, management, outcomes, cost-benefits, patient/client/service user or staff or student experience, and so on. If you are searching for information, it helps to break the topic down into several aspects.

It is important to be quite clear about what you want to find out about *before you start looking in order to be more efficient with your time.*

Refine the question

Once you have identified your broad topic, you need to focus down. Try and **put your enquiry into the form of a question** that you need to answer. This means that you seek an answer to a specific question from the literature, rather than seeking information about the entire topic. There are many approaches you can take when you **begin to define the question**. Sometimes, what you need to search for is not immediately clear and it might help to think around the topic. You could:

- Think through/reflect on your practice to isolate what really concerns you or note where there have been differences in approaches to a clinical or professional problem.
- Talk to experts.
- Brainstorm ideas with colleagues.
- Use a spider diagram or mind map.
- Carry out a quick initial database search using only one or two keywords.
- Use a search engine to see broadly what terms/subjects come up. Google Scholar can be a good place to start [http://scholar.google.co.uk/], as it is more specific and you can set filters by date, etc.
- Look in the contents page of journals specific to your specialty or the index of textbooks on the subject you are interested in for ideas on what are the key or current issues.

Examples from practice

Example 1: If you are searching for information regarding the attitudes of occupational therapists to dementia, you need to select this professional group and also specify that you are exploring attitudes, not the effectiveness of interventions.

Example 2: If you are looking for evidence about the outcomes of children at risk who were taken out of the family home, you need to look specifically at these children rather than children at risk who were not removed from the home.

Example 3: If you are wondering why your patient's leg ulcer is not responding to the treatment you are providing and you have heard that using Manuka honey might be effective in the healing process, you might want to look specifically at the effectiveness of Manuka honey.

In addition to focusing down on a specific question, it is also useful to consider exactly what type of evidence will help you address your research question. In Chapter 3, we discussed how different problems need different types of evidence and you need to be clear about what you are looking for.

Examples from practice

Example 4: If you want to know whether or not an intervention or therapy works, you need to look for RCTs or reviews of these studies in the first instance.

Example 5: If you want to know about a patient's or client's experience with a particular condition or situation, you could look for qualitative or phenomenological studies or reviews of these studies in the first instance.

Focusing and structuring your question

Using PICOT (or PICO)

When trying to choose your research question, consider using the acronym **PICOT**. Note that the letters that form PICOT have different meanings depending on whether you are looking for quantitative or qualitative research. These are outlined below. You may also come across the acronym PICO, which has the same meaning but omits the final stage. Fineout-Overholt and Johnston (2005) and Stillwell et al. (2010) suggest the following stages when defining a question, with the letters 'I' and 'C' having different meanings depending on the type of research you are looking for:

Standard PICOT	Qualitative PICOT
Population	**P**opulation
Intervention	**I**ssue
Comparison	**C**ontext
Outcome	**O**utcome
Time	**T**ime

These can be used in any order in your written question and are explained as follows:

Population, people or participants: You need to consider the people you wish to study and what characteristics they might have in common, such as gender, age, condition, problem, location, and role. For example, older people in residential care, people who are homeless, mothers under 45, children who have had orthopaedic surgery, patients/clients who have accessed paramedic services for chest pain, staff who work out of hours, students who access study advice.

Intervention (for quantitative questions): This is what you wish to evaluate – it could be diagnostic, therapeutic, preventative, managerial interventions, cost-benefit, and so on.

Issue (for qualitative questions): This is the area or topic you want to know about – it may be a concept (such as hope, partnership, bereavement), a condition (such as anxiety or asthma), a service (diabetes support programme, discharge from the service), an intervention (pain control, cognitive behavioural therapy) or a situation such as domestic violence or homelessness.

Comparison/control (for quantitative questions): The comparison can be against another intervention or no intervention; comparisons can also be made against national or professional standards or guidelines.

Context (for qualitative questions): The context of the study might be where the study takes place or factors that impact on an experience.

Outcome: for quantitative studies, this needs to be measurable – physiological observations, faster, cheaper, a reduction or increase in, for example, symptoms, benefits, events, episodes, prognosis, mortality, accuracy. For qualitative studies, this is usually expressed in the words of the participants and is descriptive/interpretive (i.e. experiences, perceptions, feelings, attitudes, and so on).

Time: This may or may not be relevant; for example, three days postoperative, five hours post-intervention, within 24 hours of accessing the service.

Examples of PICOT questions (quantitative)

Does education about smoking (**intervention, I**) reduce smoking (**outcome, O**) in young people (**population, P**) in state education (**comparison, C**, if there is a control group of young persons who did not receive education) before the age of 16 (**time, T**)?

Does the use of tap water (**I**) compared with normal saline (**C**) impact on infection rates (**O**) in older people with venous leg ulcers (**P**)?

How is readmission rate (**O**) influenced by a post-discharge telephone call (**I**) two days post-discharge (**T**) compared with usual discharge (**C**) in children undergoing orthopaedic surgery (**P**)?

How does weekly (**T**) cognitive behavioural therapy (**I**) compared with anti-depressant medication (**C**) impact on depression and anxiety self-assessment scores (**O**) in women with chronic illness (**P**)?

Examples of PICOT questions (qualitative)

Why (**outcome, O**) do young people (**population, P**) in secondary education (**context, C**) start smoking (**issue, I**) before the age of 16 (**time, T**)?

What is the experience (**O**) of older women (**P**) in the community (**C**) with venous leg ulcers (**I**)?

How do women (**P**) feel (**O**) when given a diagnosis of breast cancer (**I**) when attending outpatient departments (**C**)?

What are the perceptions (**O**) of pre-registration nursing students (**P**) of self-directed learning activities (**I**) compared with lectures (**C**) in a UK university (**C**)?

What is the experience (**O**) of homeless men (**P**) regarding risk-taking behaviours (**I**) in the community (**C**)?

See Stern et al. (2014) for further examples.

Try writing both a quantitative and qualitative research question using the PICOT process on something you want to explore in your practice.

A word of caution about using PICOT: Not all questions fit into a qualitative or quantitative approach; many questions will be answered by mixed methods. However, the tool is widely used and a good way of getting you thinking about framing a focused question.

Other tools for formulating research questions

A variety of different formulas are available to help focus a research question. Note that one is not necessarily better than another; it depends on your question. Booth (2016) has summarized some of the available tools as outlined below:

Notation	Components
3WH	What (topical), Who (population), When (temporal), How (methodological)
BeHEMoTh	Behaviour, Health context, Exclusions, Models or Theories
CIMO	Context, Intervention, Mechanisms, Outcomes
ECLIPSe	Expectations (improvement, innovation or information), Client group (recipients of service), Location (where service is housed), Impact (what change in service and how measured), Professionals involved, Service
PEICO(S)	Person, Environment, Intervention, Comparison, Outcomes, (Stakeholders)
PICO	Patient/Population, Intervention, Comparison, Outcomes
PICo	Population, phenomenon of Interest, Context
PICOC	Patient/Population, Intervention, Comparison, Outcomes, Context
PICOS	Patient/Population, Intervention, Comparison, Outcomes, Study type
SPICE	Setting, Perspective, Intervention/phenomenon of Interest, Comparison, Evaluation
SPIDER	Sample, Phenomenon of Interest, Design, Evaluation, Research type

Source: Booth (2016). See his open access paper for all the individual authors and references for each acronym.

Once you have identified what you are trying to find out, you need to consider what evidence will enable you to answer the question. While appreciating which research approaches are most likely to be relevant to answering your research question, you are advised to remain open-minded at this stage about the inclusion of all types of information if they are relevant to your research question.

Searching for relevant evidence

Once you have established the specific topic or question you want to address (***research question***), you need to develop an effective approach to your search (***search strategy***) that will enable you to identify and locate the widest range and most relevant publications within your time and financial limitations.

The importance of a comprehensive approach to searching for literature

 If you are comprehensive or systematic in your approach to searching for literature, you are likely to access the best available evidence. If you do not adopt a systematic approach, you are likely to access a random selection of literature.

What's wrong with Google? Internet search engines such as Google are **not** specific enough to search effectively, although they may give you some ideas of language terms used. This is why you need to access a **subject-specific search engine or database**.

- A literature search that is approached systematically is very different from one that is approached in a haphazard manner!
- A thorough and comprehensive search strategy will help to ensure that you identify all the key literature/texts and research on your topic.
- If you are using the information to share with others or in your writing, then documenting your stated strategy will ensure that those who access your evidence know what you looked for, what was included and excluded, and where you searched.

 Think how you might have accessed literature in the past for your learning and for your practice and consider the pros and cons of those approaches.

You may have found literature in your workplace from a search engine or website or obtained it from colleagues. Or you might have carried out a quick search and used the first thing you found. Some examples of information sources that are 'easy to access' but which may not give you a comprehensive account of evidence in the area include:

- Newspapers and other forms of media, including social media
- Websites focusing on health and social care
- Internet search engines such as Google
- Lectures and lecture notes
- Lecturers or practice assessor/mentors
- Colleagues in your professional practice area
- Journals to which your workplace/learning institution subscribes.

Although in fast-paced situations with little time you may draw on some of these sources, where a situation or issue is likely to reoccur, it is better to undertake a more thorough search.

Potential problems with haphazard/casual approaches to finding literature

- It could be out of date
- It could be biased
- You may miss out on finding key literature
- It may not be the best available evidence for the question you have
- Contradictory literature may be out there
- It may present only one aspect of the complete picture
- Harder-to-find literature may be really useful in answering your question
- Your conclusions are likely to be inaccurate.

Elsewhere we discuss the difference between information that is readily available and information that is the best available (Aveyard et al. 2015). You can see here the limitations of relying on haphazard or casual approaches to finding and using evidence – you will not find a comprehensive or full range of evidence on the topic you are interested in, however useful it is to get ideas from journals that you come across in the office, department, etc. There is likely to be far more evidence available and what you have may be 'just the tip of the iceberg'.

For a step-by-step guide to constructing a search strategy and searching for evidence, see Aromataris and Riitano (2014). You are likely to find database search guides posted on university or health and social care library websites if you have access to these.

How to develop an effective search strategy

The six steps in developing a search strategy are:

1 Be clear about the focus of your work – have a clear research question.
2 Identify your key terms, phrases, and alternative words (synonyms).
3 Define the inclusion and exclusion criteria.
4 Undertake a comprehensive search by selecting a relevant professional database, using your keywords or phrases, truncating and using Boolean operators, and focusing your search using inclusion and exclusion criteria.
5 Record your search strategy.
6 Manage and store your literature effectively.

Let us now look at each of these steps in turn.

Be clear about the focus of your literature search

If you articulate your focus at the beginning of the search process, this will help to keep you on track. State your enquiry clearly as a question as discussed above. It is important to ensure that you only search for information that is relevant to the research question as it is very easy to get sidetracked. Use one of the acronyms such as PICOT or PICO as described above to form a clear question.

Identify your keywords or key phrases

Once you have articulated the focus of your literature search using a question, you need to identify some keywords or phrases that you can use to search for literature. You will use these when you perform your search using databases, and identifying keywords or phrases within your question in the first instance will help you clarify the purpose of your search. The databases you use retrieve information by **keywords** and it is important to identify these in advance. You need to think laterally when you do this – think of the different ways in which your topic could be referred to and identify the keywords that you think are likely to represent your topic. Google, Wikipedia or a profession-specific website can help you to do this, as you will see the different ways that your topic is discussed and the phrases that are used. You can also use the **thesaurus** component, **subject index** or **MeSH** terms or **topic tree** of a database search engine (a librarian will help you understand

and access these or increasingly they may have on-line help). These help you to identify further keywords that you may not have thought of initially. You can also refer to other published literature in the area to find out how the authors of other papers have searched using keywords. You will find that your search for evidence is not a one-off process but an evolving process that you return to and refine as your ideas develop.

- You should be as creative as possible, as the topic or question might be categorized in different ways by different researchers.
- Think of all the words that mean the same thing (use a thesaurus if you can; they are often accessible on the databases).
- Consider different spellings of the same word (both British and American English) and how word endings can vary – children/child/children's (see below).
- Consider abbreviations and the use of hyphens, such as HIV/H.I.V., pathophysiology/patho-physiology.
- You also need to consider whether the keywords you identify have different meanings in different countries, especially given that databases have their own biases. For example, Cumulative Index to Nursing and Allied Health Literature (CINAHL) has a strong North American bias while the British Nursing Database has a British focus – for example, family doctor, general practitioner (G.P.), primary care physician.
- Don't limit your keywords to terms that are conventional if you think literature might be indexed using different headings.
- You will find that you identify further search terms as your search progresses.

Example

Consider the way in which the term 'learning difficulties/disabilities' is used. Some people have strong feelings about which term is used. However, if you are searching for literature in this area, be careful to use every term that might have been used to index the literature or you risk omitting vital literature from your search.

Using phrases (more than one word together)

If you string two or more words together such as time management, not all databases will link them and you may find irrelevant papers about management in general rather than time management. So, in most databases, you need to put the words inside single quotation marks, 'time management'. However, the words might also appear in other combinations or different orders, in which case you may want to have them as separate keywords and combine them with AND (see below), which would find time management but also research that discussed management of time. You may need to use trial and error to find out which approach finds the most relevant research.

Define your inclusion and exclusion criteria

Inclusion and exclusion criteria enable you to identify the literature that addresses your research question and to reject that which does not. Once you have identified your key terms, you need to identify inclusion and exclusion criteria that will assist you in selecting appropriate literature for your topic. While inclusion and exclusion criteria are generally used by those undertaking a search as part of a larger more formal literature review, the principles of including relevant and excluding irrelevant literature apply to every literature search. The criteria you develop will be guided by the wording of your research question and your focus. Unless your question clearly indicates otherwise, you will likely look for primary research or literature reviews in the first instance. You should be able to justify why you have chosen the inclusion and exclusion criteria, which ought to be determined by the needs of the question you wish to answer rather than your own convenience. For example, it would not be appropriate to include studies that are only available electronically if a hard paper copy of an article you require is available in the local library.

Example of inclusion criteria

- Primary research directly related to the topic
- English language only
- Published literature only
- 2012 onwards
- In a particular setting or a particular population or age range.

Example of exclusion criteria

- Primary research not directly related to the topic area
- Non-English language
- Unpublished research
- Pre-2012
- Not in a particular setting or with a particular population.

Should I limit my search for practical reasons?

In an ideal world, you would be able to search and locate all the information that is relevant to your specific topic and/or the question you wish to address. However, some of your criteria will be set for practical reasons, such as time and resources.

Example

Practicalities might mean you have to limit your search to recent literature and omit unpublished literature from your search. Neither of these restrictions is ideal and you might lose relevant literature – there might be a piece of work that is highly relevant to your review but which was published before the date restrictions you set.

If you set **time restrictions** to your search for literature, you could miss key documents, although they might be referred to in other published research. You should not limit your search to accessing electronic **full text availability**, because even if it is difficult to physically visit your library, most libraries will offer a photocopying or inter-library loan service.

Should I limit my search to published literature only?

Again, in an ideal world, you would seek to access all available literature on your topic or research question. There might be a lot of 'hidden' evidence about your topic that remains unpublished, called **grey literature**. Non-academic journals might also be referred to as grey literature and other sources such as policies also fall into this category. As a new researcher or someone who is starting out in professional life, you are unlikely to look for grey literature.

Undertake a comprehensive search

Once you have identified your question, keywords or phrases, and inclusion and exclusion criteria, you are ready to begin searching for literature/evidence. This is important because it will help you identify the 'best available' evidence for your academic studies and for practice.

There are five main ways of searching for literature. These are:

- Electronic searching using computer-held databases
- Searching reference lists of articles you already have (called snowballing)

- Hand searching relevant journals specific to the research topic or using electronic journal searching
- Contacting authors directly
- Searching national policy/guidelines or professional body websites.

Electronic databases

Searching for literature has become a much easier and more efficient process with the advent of electronic databases. If you have recently visited your local academic or professional library, you will be aware that this has had an enormous impact on the ways in which we search for information. In the past (when the authors were students), reviewing the literature meant having to search through bound volumes of subject-indexed references in which previously published literature was categorized under various keywords. Many of these were only updated on a yearly basis. Thus when conducting a search, anything published within the previous year was often unobtainable. Nowadays, most of the information you need is accessible through one of many electronic databases.

Three types of database are relevant when conducting a literature search:

1 Databases of systematic reviews
2 Subject-specific databases
3 Journal databases.

Databases of systematic reviews

It is a good idea to start searching a database of systematic reviews because there may have already been a comprehensive, high-quality systematic search carried out on your research question and you will save considerable time and effort. The Cochrane Library or Campbell Collaboration are good places to start, but remember that these databases' main focus is on systematic reviews of effectiveness.

Systematic reviews of qualitative research or qualitative evidence synthesis are increasingly recognized as having value (Finfgeld-Connett and Johnson 2013; Booth 2016). However, you may need to use a professional subject-specific database to access them.

Subject-specific databases

Subject-specific databases (e.g. MEDLINE) will contain references relevant to your topic of interest and allow you to search for that information, normally in the form of published academic papers (reviews, research or articles). These databases are compiled as follows: published papers are scrutinized and allocated keywords, which are then indexed. This index of keywords is then stored by the database. When you come to search the database, you enter your keywords and the database produces a list of references of the papers it holds that have been allocated your keyword. Normally, the reference is given in the form of name, date of publication, title of publication, title of journal in which the information is held, and possibly the abstract of the paper. As an added bonus, some databases provide a link to an electronic copy of the full text version of the paper; if not, you can use the electronic journal databases described below.

Journal databases

Journal databases are useful when you know exactly what you are looking for and have the information (including volume and issue number) for a particular journal article. You can locate the journal you need and from there you can locate the particular paper you are looking for. It is usually organized via date, volume number, and issue number, allowing you to access the electronic copy of the paper. It is important to note that the electronic journal database should not be used to search for what is written on your topic (subject-specific databases are better for this) but is useful to locate the sources identified from the subject-specific databases.

Getting started using databases

Identify which relevant databases you are able to access. Various health and social care databases will be available through professional websites, university or organizational libraries to which you belong. Different databases access literature from different countries or groups of countries or focus on specific specialties or interest areas. You need to ensure you use an appropriate one.

- Find out if you need a password to access a database and, if you do, set one up. Your librarian will help with this.
- Familiarize yourself with the way in which each database works, as all databases operate differently – do not assume that commands you use for one database will be understood by another.
- Access any help sheets or online tutorials or attend a training session on searching.

A selection of commonly held databases for health and social work

(Note: your own library may have others)

AMED: allied health including occupational therapy, physiotherapy, complementary therapy, and palliative care

ASSIA: Applied Social Sciences Indexes and Abstracts

Autism Data: open access database of over 18,500 published research papers, books, articles, and videos on autism

British Nursing Database: information about nursing, midwifery, and community health care, mainly from UK journals

Campbell Collaboration: systematic reviews of the effects of social interventions, such as education, crime and justice, and social welfare. An American database freely available on and off campus

CINAHL: nursing and allied health care from North America and Europe

CIRRIE: Center for International Rehabilitation Research Information and Exchange database

Cochrane Library: systematic reviews of evidence for the effectiveness of treatments

DARE: Database of Abstracts of Reviews of Effects – abstracts of systematic reviews covering effects of interventions. Note that you need to tick the box to restrict your search to DARE

DUETs: Database of Uncertainties about the Effects of Treatments

HMIC: non-clinical topics, including inequalities in health and user involvement, health services and hospital administration, management and policy

MEDLINE: connect via Ebsco, PubMed or Web of Knowledge. Extensive medical and nursing database

NICE Clinical Knowledge Summaries: evidence-based information on common conditions managed in primary care

OpenGREY: open access to SIGLE bibliographical references of reports and other grey literature produced in Europe

OTSeeker: abstracts of systematic reviews and randomized controlled trials relevant to occupational therapy

PEDRO: physiotherapy evidence database

PsycINFO: psychology, psychiatry, child development, psychological aspects of illness and treatment

PubMed: extensive medical, biomedical, and nursing database. Freely available on and off campus

Rehabdata: disability and rehabilitation – hosted by the US National Rehabilitation Information Center

Social Care Online: social and community care, includes Department of Health circulars

Social Services Abstracts: abstracts from journal articles on social work, welfare, and policy

Sociological Abstracts: sociology and political theory

Source: management and practice of primary health care and disability in developing countries

TRIP medical database: evidence-based medicine and healthcare resources on the web

Web of Science: includes Science Citation Index and Social Sciences Citation Index

ZETOC: the British Library electronic table of contents. Covers about 20,000 current journals and conference proceedings in many key subject areas

Source: Oxford Brookes University Library [http://www.brookes.ac.uk/library/subject-help/health-and-social-work/databases-for-health-and-social-work/; accessed March 2017].

For further critical evaluation, see Briscoe and Cooper (2014) who compare the British Nursing Index (now called the British Nursing Database) and CINAHL. Bramer et al. (2016) compare searches for 120 systematic reviews in Embase, MEDLINE, and Google Scholar. They conclude that Google Scholar should not be used on its own for a search of systematic reviews; other databases need also to be searched. Wright et al. (2015) discuss the value of the CINAHL database when searching for systematic reviews of qualitative studies. In relation to social work, McGinn et al. (2016) found that database performance was unpredictable and assert the importance of using a variety of resources when searching for social work-related material. They discuss other approaches such as using concept groups and search formulae, and found that two databases are most successful for social work issues: Social Services Abstracts (SSA) and PsycINFO.

Access your own academic or professional electronic library and identify which databases are relevant to your profession and interests and see if they have any helpful guides.

Boolean operators. AND, OR, and NOT are called **Boolean operators**. You should use the **AND/OR** commands in your search strategy as appropriate.

> **OR** ensures that **one term or another** is selected. Use of OR enables you to search for all the synonyms or words that mean the same thing. If you do not use the available range of ORs, you are likely to miss papers that have used alternative keywords.

> **AND** ensures that **each** term you have entered is searched for. Use of AND enables you to combine your searches. This will not only reduce the number of hits you get, but make them more relevant because each term must be included in the article for it to be recognized.

If you keep getting results that are not useful, you should seek help from a librarian or colleague.

Truncation. There is also the '*' **facility**, which enables you to identify all possible endings of the key term you write. You need to identify (try underlining) the 'root' of the word – i.e. the part of the word that doesn't change – and put the asterisk after that last common letter. For example, <u>child</u>* will identify articles containing child, <u>children</u>, children's, and so on.

A **wildcard** replaces one or more letters in a word when there is more than one spelling. For example, for woman/women the wildcard is 'Wom?n', or to find pediatrics (US spelling) or paediatrics (UK spelling) use 'pe?diatrics'.

You may find it useful to type your search as several 'search strings'. You can then 'cut and paste' them into several databases. For example, experience OR perception* OR perceive* OR feel*.*

Using the table on p. 123 will help you to structure your search using all the Boolean operators (AND, OR, and truncation). A blank copy of the table you can use as a template follows the example.

1 Insert your main keywords (from your research question) across the top, the most important ones first. You can add extra rows if you need to.
2 Then in each column add the synonyms (words that mean the same as the keyword). Think of alternative spellings; if there are plurals or alternative endings, use truncation; consider abbreviations and hyphens. Use 'single quote marks' for phrases to keep the words together.
3 You can then use each keyword and its synonyms as a search. For example:

Search 1: attitude* OR stigma* OR approach* OR opinion* OR view*
Search 2: student* or baccalaureate* OR undergraduate* OR pre-registration OR pre-qualifying

4 You can then combine the searches one at a time. For example: Search 1 AND Search 2 or Search 1 AND Search 2 AND Search 3, or even Search 1 AND Search 3, and so on depending on what provides the most relevant resources.
5 You can then narrow down by dates. Ideally, you want to find few enough references so that you can review ALL the abstracts.

See later in the chapter for more ideas on search techniques and common mistakes made.

1 Search 1 Keyword		2 Search 2 Keyword		3 Search 3 Keyword		4 Search 4 Keyword
Attitude*	AND	Student*	AND	Nurse (or state other profession)	AND	'Human immunodeficiency virus'
Or		Or		Or		Or
Stigma*		Baccalaureate*		Nurs*		HIV
Or		Or				Or
Approach*		Undergraduate*				H.I.V.
Or		Or				Or
Opinion*		Pre-registration				'Acquired immunodeficiency syndrome'
Or		Or				Or
View*		Pre-qualifying				AIDS
Source: adapted from Oldershaw (2009).						

Identify search terms for a question you have using the template below (you can add rows or columns if you need to).

Underline each keyword or 'phrase', remembering that the words in each column should have the same meaning. Use truncation (*) to get plurals or alternative endings. You may need to add columns or rows.

1 Search 1 Keyword		2 Search 2 Keyword		3 Search 3 Keyword		4 Search 4 Keyword
	AND		AND		AND	
Or		Or		Or		Or
Or		Or		Or		Or
Or		Or		Or		Or
Or		Or		Or		Or

In a large Cochrane systematic review, Wolfenden et al. (2016) identified 110 search terms.

Most databases default to searching with the keywords they used to classify the individual papers (this is usually in a drop-down menu at the side of the search box).

In many databases, you can specify whether you would like to search throughout the whole article *(text) for the term, or whether you want to limit your search to the* abstract *(the short summary) or just the* title.

- If you limit your search to just the title, you may exclude a lot of references that might be relevant to you, as some titles will not use the key terms you have identified.

- Searching the abstract for your keywords and their synonyms generally will find a manageable amount of results (for example, if you do not find enough when searching using the title or if you find too many when searching the whole article/text).
- If you search through the whole article (text) for your keyword, you are likely to be overwhelmed with literature and will need to use further exclusion criteria to narrow your results down.
- Limiting your search to the abstract is likely to be a suitable compromise, as the keywords you have selected should be evident in the abstracts of relevant papers.
- If you get very few articles based on a less common or unusual keyword, you may want to search the whole article.

You are likely to need to refine your search strategy as you progress. You will find that you will develop new ideas as you undertake the search process. You might find, for example, a key theme is called by a different name or phrase that you had not previously thought of. Be aware of this and be prepared to search using new and different keywords or phrases.

Once you have identified the key literature on your topic using one database, you could repeat the search using another database. This will depend on the requirements of your search. If you find that the same references are duplicated, then you can be confident that your strategy is well focused and that you are accessing the relevant literature on your topic. You might feel it is appropriate to scale down your search using limiters such as date.

Getting help

Your subject librarian at your university or place of work will be happy to guide you. Your local library is likely to provide tutorials, video guidance or help sheets on searching for evidence. When you get started, you will find academic journals relating to a very wide range of professional interests. Some journals are generic to the interests of one professional group – for example, the *Journal of Clinical Nursing* or the *British Journal of Occupational Therapy* – whereas others are specialist journals that focus on a particular area of professional interest – for example, *Addiction*. Academic journals contain many articles about different topics related to the overall subject addressed by the journal.

Journals often contain a mixture of research, literature reviews, and discussion/opinion articles, which we discuss in more depth later in the book.

Remember . . .

- Searching for literature is time-consuming and requires skill – you are advised not to leave it until the last minute before you start your search.
- If you do not have any 'hits' from your search, you need to keep searching with different keywords until you identify literature that is linked to your topic area. If you have too many hits, you will need to refocus your search.
- Keep a record of the search terms you have used and the results of these searches.
- If new references are constantly being thrown up, you will need to continue searching until later searches reveal little or no new information.

Why are electronic searches not 100% effective?

 Despite advances in electronic searching, computerized search tools are not 100% effective and will fail to identify some of the relevant literature on your topic.

Electronic searches are not 100% effective because:

- Some relevant literature might have been categorized using different keywords and thus cannot be identified by one particular search strategy.
- The topic you are looking for may be mentioned in several papers but not to a great extent and therefore was not indexed when these papers were entered on to the database. This means that the papers will not be recognized by the database when you search for this topic.
- You may have only searched within the title of articles and the title may be misleading.

Authors who use imaginative or humorous titles for their work run the risk that it will not be found by others conducting a search on the same topic. Although using various keywords will help identify literature that is not identified on the first search, it is still possible for literature to remain unidentified even though it is highly relevant to addressing the research question.

Is searching for evidence an art or a science?

We have emphasized that searching for evidence will never be a one-off process. You need to ensure you have conducted a thorough search of the available evidence and continue to update and refine your search. The more you search, the more you will begin to develop instinct and experience about where to search and what terms are used around your subject matter. **Knowledge of your subject matter** will certainly help with this.

Example

An inexperienced searcher may search for 'use of gloves AND aprons' in infection control. A more experienced individual will realize that it is better to search under the terms 'universal OR standard precautions' rather than search for individual protective equipment.

Thus you should regard searching for evidence as both a science and an art. Searching should be regarded as a science, because we encourage you to undertake a **methodological and comprehensive** approach to the identification of relevant evidence. Searching should also be regarded as an art because you also need to be **creative and flexible** about the way you identify relevant evidence. There are additional ways that you can search. Students are often concerned that any additional methods of searching they use will cause their search strategy to appear 'haphazard'. The key point here is, if these searches are *in addition* to a comprehensive database search, then any other references they identify can only enrich your search. However, if they are *instead* of a comprehensive database search, then the search strategy is at risk of becoming 'haphazard'.

Searching article reference lists

This is sometimes called **snowballing** (not to be confused with snowball sampling, which is a way of selecting participants for research). Once you have identified the key articles that relate to your research question, you might want to scrutinize the reference lists of those **key articles** for further references that may be relevant. You will use the same keywords and inclusion and exclusion criteria to do this, although you may come across important older key texts, which are frequently referenced but that fall outside your exclusion dates. Horsley et al. (2011) carried out a Cochrane systematic review entitled 'Checking reference lists to find additional studies for systematic reviews'. They concluded that there was some evidence to support the checking of reference lists for locating studies in systematic reviews and it would likely be useful when hand searching or searching databases is difficult. It would therefore seem prudent that authors of reviews check reference lists to supplement their search.

Hand-searching relevant journals

If you notice that many of the key articles you have identified as being relevant to your research question have been published in one or two journals, it might be useful to hand-search these journals to locate other relevant articles that have not been identified through other search strategies. Searching through the contents pages of these journals may identify other relevant material. This may also be done electronically through an A–Z of journals and selecting the relevant journal (some journal websites have archive search facilities).

Author searching/consulting experts

If you find that many of your key articles are by the same author(s), it may be useful to carry out an author search to identify whether the author(s) have published other works not identified by the electronic search. This might also lead you towards work in progress. In some specialist areas, it may be worth contacting the author directly to see if they are aware of any other sources. **Experts** in a clinical or professional area may have attended conferences or be involved in projects that address your issue or question. Contacting them directly may highlight new sources. If they are helpful, it is considered polite to share your findings with them once your research is complete. If your topic includes a product or service, the manufacturer/supplier may have commissioned research. However, you need to be aware of the potential bias of such research.

 Remember that it takes time and practice to become accustomed to database searching. If you are a practice assessor/mentor, ask your student to show you how to search.

Professional body or government publications

Remember that your professional body or association will have many resources and it will be useful to consult these to find additional sources of information. In health and social care, there may be government policy or legislation that can provide a useful addition to your search strategy.

Using a **combination of the above search strategies** will ensure that you have the most comprehensive search strategy and therefore the best chance of retrieving the information that is relevant to your research question.

How to use abstracts to confirm the relevance of papers

Once you have identified the literature that is relevant to you, the next step is to sort through the results list you now have and identify which references are most relevant. To do this, you **cannot rely on the title alone**. This is because the focus of the article, whether or not it is a primary research study, is often unclear from the title alone. You may also want to consider your 'hierarchy of evidence' (discussed in Chapter 4) to find the best available evidence.

The abstract *will provide a summary of the content of the article, in particular whether it is a research article or not.*

The abstract is often available on electronic databases such as CINAHL and MEDLINE. However, abstracts can themselves be unreliable sources for determining the exact focus of a paper, and you might find that you miss relevant literature if you discard a paper because of the information contained in the abstract. However, given that you are unlikely to be able to access in full each paper you identify from an electronic search, you will have to rely on the abstract to determine whether or not the paper will address your research question. If you cannot tell from the abstract, you will need to access the paper in order to do this.

> **Common mistakes when searching a database**
>
> **Start to search too early** – without having a clear focus or question, e.g. search for dementia instead of 'how do carers of adults with dementia manage stress?'

Not selecting the most appropriate databases – you need to think about and read information about each database, e.g. Cochrane may be best for finding out about effectiveness of interventions, PsychINFO may be best to understand the psychological impact of an issue or condition.

Putting the truncation symbol * in the wrong place – the * symbol should be used at the end of the common letters of a word, for example, diabet*, the common letters of the words diabetes, diabetic.

Not understanding the Boolean operator 'OR' – 'OR' is used to search for **all words** that could have the same meaning, or synonyms. You would search for these all together to ensure you don't miss out on a key source that uses an alternative term. This will increase the hits you get (you can reduce this number later with the AND command). You can look at keywords on the papers you find that are relevant (often on the first page of articles) or you can use MeSH terms (usually an option on the database) and ask other people for help.

Selecting too many keywords – once you have your topic and you have selected the most important keywords and combined them using the Boolean operator AND, you should decide which are crucial to what you want to find out. For example, bold font in the following question: 'What is **the experience** of **teenagers** with **depression** attending **outpatient clinics**?' If you have a lot of keywords, you may want to **start searching with the two most common** keywords (and their synonyms) and then add in the others to narrow your search down further, in this case **teenagers** and **depression.** You do this by typing in Keyword 1 (and all its synonyms) AND Keyword 2 (and all its synonyms). You can then add AND Keyword 3 (and all its synonyms), and so on. You may also want to try different combinations, e.g. Keywords 1 and 3 or 2 and 4, etc.

Not finding all the keywords – you may need to think of alternative spellings (sometimes American and British English differ). You can use a wildcard which is a '?' in place of an unknown letter, for example, for pediatric* or paediatric* you could put p?ediatric*. Think about abbreviations too, e.g. HIV/H.I.V.

Not using enough or too many limiters – if you have combined your keywords (and their synonyms) and still have lots of hits (perhaps more than 100), you need to add some limiters (these can be your exclusion criteria) such as **by Date:** you could limit to the previous 10 years initially, then, if still too many, the last 5 years. For rapidly changing and recent topics, you could limit to the last 2 or 3 years. Remember to look in reference lists for any KEY or SEMINAL (still considered important, but older) papers – they are often the ones most referenced by other people. This could be research or theory that has not been replaced or repeated. For short assignments, you could limit by **full text accessibility**, but for more substantail work such as a dissertation, you would be expected to get the hard copy of key papers.

Searching the 'whole text' for 'common' keywords and getting too many hits! – if the keyword you are searching for is likely to be mentioned in a broad range of subjects, say, hand-washing (even when the paper is not about hand-washing), you should narrow it down by searching in the **abstract** or, if it is still widely mentioned, in the **title**. For example, if you are looking for 'observations', a paper may not be about observations but reports that a patient/client was observed.

Remember to PLAN the search before you access the databases.

Getting hold of sources

Don't be put off if there is no obvious link to a pdf file of the paper you want on the database results. Not all databases include a full text link. Follow the instructions on the database for the best way to access the paper.

The references you have found are likely to be in journals, books, and other publications. You can **find journal articles** in a variety of ways:

- Access the journal directly via their website or sometimes a search engine on the Internet. Many publications now have 'open access' papers that are free to download, sometimes for a limited period.
- Access an academic or professional electronic library and search e-journals, using the Internet, with a password supplied by your librarian.
- Access the paper copies (often referred to as hard copies) in your library.

Try to access training on using your local library (especially from a subject specialist) to help you locate publications.

- Most university and workplace libraries will have many journals accessible as '**full-text**' electronically and you will find that you can locate and download many articles without leaving your computer. Sometimes this is indicated by a small symbol. **You will need a password to access these**. There is sometimes – but not always – a link from the database to the full-text article in the electronic library.
- You are strongly advised to familiarize yourself with the journals to which you have easy access through your local library. Some libraries will have a subject-specific catalogue. University libraries may have fewer clinical sources than a health or social care library, so it is worth checking both if you have access.
- If the reference you require is not available full-text electronically, then you will need to access the bound volumes available as hard copies in the library.
- If the references are not available electronically or in bound volumes in your local library, you will need to either arrange to visit another library or arrange an **inter-library loan**. This will bear a small cost and be time-consuming, so you need to decide whether it is worth doing so.
- It may be worth trying a general Internet search or consult https://scholar.google.co.uk/ for the article, as increasingly they may be posted on websites. Do make sure it is the complete original article (best as a pdf file) and that it has not been summarized or altered.

Strengths and limitations of your search strategy

Clearly, if you are doing a more detailed systematic review, you need to make every effort to retrieve all the articles relevant to your study. When undertaking a smaller-scale literature search, you do not need to go to the same lengths to retrieve literature, although of course the more comprehensive the search, the better. Overall, your search will be more comprehensive the more effort you expend in locating all the references that are central to your question.

Some potential limitations of a search

Experience of the researchers

If you are doing a project by yourself, you are unlikely to have the same skills and resources as a team of people working together. Those working together can share ideas, read abstracts and papers together, and so on. If you are a novice researcher, you are more likely to miss sources than a more experienced researcher.

Potential bias

You should identify any potential bias of the sources you used – if you have been unable to track down certain sources, you should acknowledge this. If you have limited your sources by accessibility, then this should be acknowledged, or if papers you cite are sponsored by a company or organization, which might have influenced the results, again acknowledge this.

Apparent lack of relevant research

This is often very frustrating if you have undertaken a systematic approach to your search yet still fail to find literature. Don't worry though, as this is still a useful finding. In fact, many Cochrane reviews conclude that there is not enough high-quality research on a topic. What you can do next is to consider if you could search within a wider context or population group and transfer that learning to your original question. For evidence-based practice, knowing there is little or no research on a topic means we can make our decisions using previous experience, reflection, and clinical/professional judgement, as discussed in Chapter 1. A single source of evidence that has not been 'judged' or appraised for its quality is generally not enough. We will consider this aspect of evidence further later in the book.

Document your search strategy

It will be helpful if you keep a record of your search strategy, the keywords or combinations of words that you used, and the number of hits, so that you can demonstrate a systematic approach.

See the table on p. 123 and consider using each of the columns to record the number of hits and then combine them to produce your final search results. This may be especially useful for academic assignments or if you are sharing the results of your search with other professionals/colleagues as evidence for your practice or if required as evidence for maintaining your professional registration. The reader should clearly be able to see how you refined your search and got to the final ones that you reviewed. A systematic search should be able to be repeated by someone else who would find the exact same papers.

Example

If you are searching for primary research articles concerned with partnership working in social care, you might initially undertake two basic searches and then combine these searches:

Database: CINAHL 2008 – Search term: partnership* – Total number of hits: 30,000

Database: CINAHL 2008 – Search term: partnership* AND social care* – Total number of hits: 15,000

You can then demonstrate how you expanded this search to include other terms and then combine this search with another search in order to obtain a more manageable number of hits.

It might also be useful to demonstrate the success of your search strategy and which searches yielded the best results. It is also useful to state what type of literature your hits included, if you can determine this from the abstracts available. If you are searching for articles of primary research but have failed to do so, you can document this.

Tips for documenting your search strategy

- Remember that the aim is to demonstrate how you undertook a **systematic approach** to your searching.
- Discuss **the approach** you took to develop an effective search strategy.
- **Keep a record** of all the search terms used so that you can provide evidence of your approach if asked.
- Keep a record of the **other approaches** you employed to search for literature.
- Be able to comment on the **effectiveness** of the approaches you used. For example, if electronic searching did not yield as many hits as you had hoped, discuss why this might have been.
- Make every effort to **obtain** relevant literature.
- It is more accurate to write '*I did not find any literature on X*' than categorically '*there is no literature . . .*'

 We recommend that you avoid statements in your writing that declare that there is no literature on a particular topic and state instead, if asked, that no literature was identified *on the topic in question.*

Manage and store your literature effectively

Remember to:

• Back up (save) all your records and keep them in a safe place throughout your search process. Save files with the date and time to avoid mixing up versions.
• Keep records on more than one site or in 'the Cloud' (what if your computer was stolen or there was a fire?) and consider emailing a copy of your reference list to yourself.
• If you are using full text electronic copies of articles, create a folder so they are kept together.
• Write references down in full every time you read something useful. It is very frustrating to have to track down page numbers or editions of references you have mislaid.
• Consider using a reference manager such as ENDNOTE, which will hold all your references electronically and produce a reference list in the format you require.
• A clear record/table or search strategy sheet should show how you got to the articles you are using to underpin your conclusions and so it could be repeated by someone else who would identify the same articles.

In summary

You should now be aware of the importance of a systematic search strategy. This will ensure that you access a comprehensive range of literature that is relevant to your question. The use of inclusion and exclusion criteria will help to ensure that the literature identified is relevant to your review question. The need to combine electronic searching of relevant databases with additional strategies such as hand-searching journals and examining reference lists has been discussed. You need to understand that electronic searching can never be fully comprehensive and that 'snowballing', using many different strategies to identify literature, will usually be the most effective way of achieving the most comprehensive literature search. At the end of the search process, you will achieve a manageable list of references that are relevant to your research question, which you will be able to locate in your academic/professional library.

At this point, you should be confident that you have identified the most relevant literature that will enable you to answer your research question. You should be aware of the strengths and limitations of your search strategy and be prepared to justify your approach if asked. It is now time to stand back and take a critical look at the literature you have identified. We will discuss how you can do this in the next chapter.

Key points

1 You need a focused question in order to identify your search terms.
2 It is important to identify the types of literature that will enable you to answer your research question.
3 Inclusion and exclusion criteria should be specific to your question.
4 The literature search strategy should incorporate a variety of approaches, including electronic searching, hand-searching, and reference list searching.

Quiz questions

1 Why is it sometimes useful to restrict your use of the AND command when searching for literature?
2 Why is database searching not sufficient for a comprehensive search?
3 What is the difference between searching for a keyword in the full text of a paper compared with the title or abstract?

6 How do I know if the evidence is convincing and useful?

In previous chapters, we have addressed how you identify the type of evidence that you need and how you find it. In this chapter, we discuss how you know that you have found relevant information and how to recognize different types of evidence. We will also explore how you can tell if the information and evidence you find is of good quality.

Overall, we want you to move from a position where you would be tempted to say *'I've read this so it must be true'* to a position where you say *'I've read this – now I need to know if it is reliable'*. Specifically, we will explore:

- Definitions of critical appraisal, its importance and key terms
- How to organize and identify the type of evidence you find from your literature search
- How to judge the quality and quantity of different sources of evidence we use (critical appraisal).

What is critical appraisal?

 Critical appraisal is the structured process of examining a piece of evidence in order to determine its strengths and limitations *and therefore the* relevance or weight *it should have in addressing your research question/ argument.*

Gray and Grove describe critical appraisal as

> . . . *the systematic, unbiased, careful examination of each aspect of studies to judge their strengths, limitations, trustworthiness, meaning and applicability to practice.*
>
> (Gray and Grove 2016: 432)

What is important is that the appraiser needs to **interpret** what is read, i.e. not just accept it. This is vitally important, given the vast amount of information there is on any one topic and it illustrates the need to be both **selective and critical** of what you read. Any piece of evidence will not do – you need to make sure you have the **best available** evidence.

When you critically appraise, you **evaluate or judge the quality and usefulness** of the evidence you have. This is the case whether you are writing an essay, a dissertation or using evidence directly in practice. It is also relevant for evaluating arguments and discussion about care delivery in professional practice. We discuss this in more detail elsewhere (Aveyard et al. 2015). The evidence you use will affect the quality of your academic work or the care provided in the clinical/professional environment.

The importance of critical appraisal

The controversy surrounding the measles, mumps, and rubella (MMR) vaccination described in Chapter 4 illustrates the importance of undertaking critical appraisal of all research and other information that you encounter. The publication that sparked the controversy was published in 1998 (Wakefield et al. 1998) and the media scare is well known. It is difficult to find a better example of the need to be critical of published evidence. And in this case the evidence was published in a top-ranking journal. Any practitioner who had read Wakefield's original article could see at a glance that the evidence it provided was not strong – the research was carried out on just twelve children and the circumstances in which the research was undertaken have caused several of the authors to retract their involvement in the study.

However, none of this prevented the **media scare** that took over and there was evidence that practitioners became reluctant to administer the MMR vaccination and parents became reluctant to take their children for vaccination. A recent study by McHale et al. (2016) found that many parents still have concerns about the link between autism and the MMR vaccination. The MMR controversy illustrates the **importance of critical appraisal** of research and other information so that you can identify how strong and relevant the evidence is relating to a particular topic.

Terms for judging the quality of research

When you read about critical appraisal, you will find many terms that come up time and time again. It is important to know what these mean. Their use can vary with the type of research.

Authors of studies usually define the terms they use or include a glossary. It is important to know what we mean by these. The following terms apply to all types of research:

- ***Relevance*** *– research that can be applied to any patient or client group and context.*

- **Rigour** – *evidence that the research has been carried out in a robust manner.*
- **Reproducibility** – *the study is clearly described and could be repeated.*

The following are mainly associated with quantitative studies:

- **Bias** – *an error in the design or conduct of research that leads to a false result. For example, in an RCT you compare one treatment or intervention against another. If another aspect of care or treatment differs between the two arms of the trial and that changes the outcomes, this would be bias. This is why we try to use blinding in a trial so that this does not happen.*
- **Generalizability** – *findings of the research that can be applied to other people in other settings.*
- **Reliability** – *the same results/conclusions would be found if the research were to be repeated.*

The following are mainly associated with qualitative studies:

- **Applicability** – *can the findings of the study be used in relation to my patients/clients?*
- **Credibility** – *evidence that the results or conclusions are believable.*
- **Transferability** – *the results of the study may be transferred to another context or population.*
- **Trustworthiness** – *honest and reliable reporting of a study.*
- **Dependability** – *can you rely on the results as they are presented?*
- **Confirmability** – *could the study be repeated?*

In addition:

- **Strengths** – *the good things about the literature, in relation to the points above.*
- **Limitations or weaknesses** – *what could be criticized about the literature, in relation to the points above.*

It is considered good practice for authors to identify some of the strengths and limitations themselves.

Getting started with critical appraisal

Every time you pick up a newspaper, you probably form a judgement as to whether or not you believe what you have read; you might even wonder which sources were used to write the article. If you don't believe what you have read, you might be tempted to track down the sources upon which the article is based. Then what usually happens (well, for us anyway) is that you don't have time to research this further and you never really find out if what you read was true or not . . . Now consider the way you approach your professional reading. Just as we are sceptical about what we read in the papers, so we should be sceptical about what we read in academic journals. This is the start of **critical appraisal**.

You should also think the same way about what you hear from colleagues or practice assessors/mentors. This will be discussed in more detail in the next chapter.

Think back to how you have used literature or other forms of evidence in the past and consider the potential problems with your approach. Did you:

- *Scan read it?*
- *Use only one or two sources?*
- *Only use what agreed with the point you wanted to make?*
- *Only use readily available sources?*
- *Copy literature without really understanding it?*
- *Ignore research that didn't agree with your current practice?*
- *Just use quotes or sections that agreed with your view?*
- *Believe everything that was written without questioning the authority of the writer or the quality of the arguments or evidence?*

It is important not to fall into either of the following two categories:

1 **You accept any piece of research** or other information at face value and accept what is written without question. You may believe that a paper published in a high-quality journal or written by an expert is above critique and so do not attempt any structured appraisal of the paper.

Even a paper that is published in a reputable journal must be examined for rigour and the relevance that it has to the topic area.

2 You may interpret the term 'critical appraisal' to mean that **you must criticize and find fault** with everything that you read. Often the term

critical is interpreted to mean that unless you 'tear to pieces' what you find, you have not done your job. Although it is always possible to find faults with a piece of research, it needs to be remembered that no research is perfect. Therefore, when you look for strengths and weaknesses, remember to take a balanced approach. More credible authors may identify within their own methodology what they consider to be any weaknesses with their approach.

Access some research from a professional journal and see if you can identify any critical comment on the paper.

Many journals offer a review of the paper alongside the article or in the next issue. Try and spot how a reviewer offers both positive and negative comments on the paper.

Note that most journals use a system of peer review before they accept articles for publication. This is a process in which experts in a subject area are invited to review the academic work of another author, prior to publication in a journal. You might be tempted to think that if a paper is published in a peer-reviewed journal, you can accept it at face value, without the need to appraise it. However, peer review is not perfect. Peer-reviewed papers, however, are more likely to contain relevant and reliable evidence, so where possible try to use journals that follow a peer-review process. Sometimes corrections or amendments to a paper are printed in a later issue of the journal. In reality, the peer-review process takes place when the research paper is published. As a general rule, just as you may be more likely to take an argument more seriously if it is published in one newspaper compared with another, this is also the case with academic journals, but do exercise some caution and do use your critical appraisal skills to evaluate every paper you read.

Another point to note is that there has been a rise in scam publishers. These 'open-access' predatory publishers are a well-organized, sophisticated scam industry only interested in making money not scholarly activity (Dadkhah et al. 2015). They receive payment from authors who want to get published more quickly and with less scrutiny, According to Darbyshire et al. (2016), they 'risk the very notion of academic standards and scholarly quality as these relate to the dissemination and sharing of our research and thinking'. The International Academy of Nursing Editors (INANE) provides a list of reputable journals for nurses [available at: https://nursingeditors.com/journals-directory/] and up until January 2017 there was a more widely published list called Beall's list; however, this has now been removed (see Watson 2017). A directory of peer-reviewed open access journals is also available from the Directory of Open Access Journals (DOAJ) [see https://doaj.org/].

Access a journal's website for an overview of its publishing process and ask educationalists/senior colleagues what are considered high-quality journals in your own field.

How do you identify if you have got a research paper or review of research?

It is important that you identify what type of information you have, so that you know that you have the most appropriate information for your needs. First of all, determine whether the evidence you have is a research paper or a review of research. This is not always as easy as it sounds!

A research or review paper usually begins with a research question, hypothesis or clear aim, and has a methods section followed by results or findings and then a conclusion. There is also likely to be an abstract that is a summary of this information.

You may be lucky and find a recent, good quality systematic review but remember you still need to appraise it. If not, then you need to appraise and synthesize all the information you have found. At this point, it is normal to feel swamped by the amount of literature and perhaps the unfamiliar terms and language used in the papers you find. It will get easier the more you read and remember to look up the terms you don't understand.

Refer back to Chapter 4 or access another research textbook or glossary to find out more about the research methods that are used in the papers you have accessed.

There are many different types of research in health and social care and the format for describing the research and results will vary widely, although the fundamental features of describing the methods used to undertake the research and the research findings should be clearly described in all research papers. They may use the words study, review or mention specific types of research that you will need to look up if you are unfamiliar with them. The abstract should help you to identify if the evidence you have is a research paper or not.

Example *abstract* from a research paper (Magrunder et al. 2016)

Purpose: The purpose of this paper is to evaluate provider outcomes in response to two modes of suicide prevention training (e-learning and in-person) and a control group. The Collaborative Assessment and Management of Suicidality (CAMS) was adapted for e-learning delivery to US Veterans Administration mental health providers. Outcomes include: self-evaluated beliefs, ability, and self-efficacy in managing suicidal patients.

Design/methodology/approach: This study used a multicenter, randomized, cluster design to test the effectiveness of e-learning vs in-person conditions CAMS for changes in provider outcomes.

Findings: Survey scores showed significant improvements for both the e-learning vs control and the in-person vs control between pre-intervention and post-intervention; however, the e-learning and in-person conditions were not significantly different from each other.

Research limitations/implications: Limitations of the study include that there were drop-outs over the study period and the survey questions may not have captured all of the aspects of the CAMS training.

Practical implications: Results suggest that e-learning training modules can provide comparable outcomes to in-person training for suicide prevention.

You can see from this abstract that the paper is a research paper, reporting the findings of a randomized controlled trial. However, it is not always so easy to recognize a piece of research. For example, bear the following points in mind:

- Beware news reports of research published in the news section of journals (or the national television news) that just show headline 'high-impact' findings but omit all other findings. This is not a full report of the research but is reported on by a journalist, who may have cherry-picked what he wanted to write about. Try to obtain the original research paper.
- Beware academic writing that refers to lots of research and resembles a review of research but does not have a methods section that tells you how the review was carried out, including databases and search terms used. If you cannot see this amount of detail, then you are probably not looking at a good quality literature review. Melnyk (2016b) notes that many unsystematic reviews are published and these can mislead practitioners. She emphasizes that unsystematic reviews should not be used as a basis to change practice. Always look for a systematic review with

published methods in which the researchers tell you how they searched for the literature they include.

If you are wondering whether you have a piece of research or a systematic review of research, look for 'methods' and 'results/findings' sections. If you cannot find any, the paper is probably not research.

If you have identified research, Greenhalgh (2014) states that there are **three preliminary questions** to get you started with critical appraisal:

Question 1: What was the research question – and why was the study needed? The first sentence of a research paper should state clearly the background. For example, '*It is widely known that . . . however . . . there is a lack of clear evidence that . . .*'. There should then be a brief literature review to show awareness of what is known about the topic.

Question 2: What was the research design? You should assess if the paper is reporting from primary (*they did their own research*) or secondary sources (*they are reporting or summarizing other studies*).

Question 3: Was the research design appropriate to the question? We have discussed this in detail in Chapter 4 where we refer to the concept of 'hierarchies of evidence' and how certain types of research suit certain research questions. We also refer to the concept of developing 'your own hierarchy of evidence' (Aveyard 2014) for the information needs that you have. The main point to re-emphasize is that there is no one 'hierarchy of evidence', and the one you adopt will depend on what you need to find out.

You may find it useful to use a research textbook or glossary to look up any methods or research types you are unfamiliar with – or ask someone! You could use a health or social care **dictionary** or online **glossary:**

Some useful glossaries to help you understand research terms:

National Institute of Health research Evaluation, Trials and Studies (NETS): http://www.nets.nihr.ac.uk/glossary?result_1655_result_page=A

Social Care Institute for Excellence (SCIE): http://www.resmind.swap.ac.uk/content/00_other/glossary.htm

Cochrane glossary: http://community-archive.cochrane.org/glossary/5

CONSORT glossary: http://www.consort-statement.org/resources/glossary

---

How do you identify if you have got a discussion or opinion paper?

Discussion or opinion papers will not have the same structure as a research paper and will generally be introduced as representing the opinion of the author. Sometimes, however, there is no such introduction and the aim of the paper might not be so easy to identify. You need to read the paper closely to ascertain what the aims and purpose of the paper are. Remember that however authoritative the writer sounds, if he or she is only expressing an opinion, this evidence remains anecdotal.

It is common to come across informative papers that provide a general update about a topic. They are often written up in 'essay' style. At first glance, you might think that you have found a literature review, because such papers often refer to lots of research; however, if you look closely, the paper will not have a methods section to explain how the authors found their literature. It can be difficult to identify whether such updates have been compiled using a systematic and unbiased approach or not.

 In principle, if the paper does not include a specific question and a method stating how the literature was searched, you should not consider it to be a comprehensive review.

Such a paper will provide less strong evidence than a review that has been compiled systematically. Remember that the quality of this type of evidence will depend on the person writing the paper. Papers like this can be very useful but do not assume that an expert is using relevant evidence-based sources upon which to base his or her argument. There may be bias in the selection of the sources used.

Example of an *abstract* from a paper that is not a systematic review or research paper (SCIE 2016)

Note that there is no mention of a research design in this paper but the authors do discuss the topic.

Reports on a roundtable event, jointly hosted by the Social Care Institute for Excellence (SCIE) and Madano, to *discuss* the impact of the Care Act on the voluntary, community and social enterprise (VCSE) sector and the new opportunities it offers. Issues *discussed* include: the opportunities and challenges of the prevention and well-being agenda, what the Care Act means for the type of services that the VCSE sector provides, what the Care Act means for commissioning practice, what enables greater engagement between the VCSE sector and others and the barriers to greater engagement. Key messages from the *discussion* include: the importance of co-production and design; for the VCSE sector to work together to develop a holistic response, rather than creating a competitive culture; for commissioners and providers to understand where preventative care 'fits'; cross-discipline working which focuses on outcomes; and the need for real cultural and behavioural change, with a willingness for commissioners and the VCSE sector to work together.

Getting to know your literature

The next thing to do is to **become familiar** with the literature you have got. Read and **re-read** the material you have so that you become familiar with it. Check that you are confident that you know which type of evidence you have: research, discussion or other evidence. At this point, you should be able to discuss with confidence the content of your papers.

Read a study or review and see if you can discuss it in detail with someone else without referring back to the paper or at least with minimal reference!

Relevance or applicability of the research

Making sense of each individual paper you come across is therefore very important and will enable you to make important assessments as to the relevance of a paper to your topic of study as well as identifying its strengths and limitations – and therefore the impact that the paper will have on addressing what you are trying to find out.

At first glance, a research paper might appear to address your research question directly, whereas on closer inspection you realize that the scope of the paper is very different from what your initial assessment had led you to believe and in fact has only indirect relevance to your research question.

You might find that although the context of the paper is relevant to your research question, the methods adopted were poorly carried out and you are less confident in the results of the study as a result.

Group your literature together so that you have all the qualitative research papers in one pile, the quantitative papers in another, discussion and opinion in another, and so on. Be aware that some may comprise

Table 6.1 Sample table for helping you summarize the papers identified by your search

Authors' names	Aims of review/study or research question	Journal	Type of evidence	Strengths	Limitations	Main findings
Smith and Brown (2017)	They have three clear objectives . . .	*Journal of Applied Social Work*: peer reviewed	Systematic review	Clear methodology Good quality studies . . .	It is 6 years old and things may have changed	They found that . . .
Carter and White (2016)	Vague statement . . . differs from the abstract	*International Journal of Physiotherapy*	Randomized controlled trial	Good sample size, wide range of participants	Doesn't discuss ethical issues/ consent or how the authors carried out blinding	Clear statistical significance in main finding statement . . .

mixed methods. It could be that you have several studies of a single type of research, a combination of qualitative and quantitative research, maybe some systematic reviews, and other non-research information, such as discussion and opinion articles.

Activity: you may want to organize a table or index cards to help you sort out the information you have. Consider using colour highlighters or Post-it™ notes to help with this. Fill in what you can and then, as you develop your appraisal skills, add more.

You may find a **table format** helpful to **summarize** what you have found. If you have been working through this book systematically, you should be able to fill in all the categories except the strengths and limitations, which we address next in the chapter (see Table 6.1).

When you have done this, you will be able to **select the correct appraisal tool** for the type of research you have identified. In the next section we discuss the use of critical appraisal tools in more detail. It is important to note that before you use a tool, you need to be familiar with the research approach that you come across. A critical appraisal tool will not help you understand the research used in the paper – it merely prompts you to ask relevant questions of the paper. Before you appraise a paper, **you need to be familiar with the research methodology** used in that paper. Therefore, if you are uncertain as to what constitutes good quality research for a particular research method, read more widely about that particular research approach.

General critical appraisal tools

Critical appraisal tools are checklists to help you ask questions of the evidence you have in order to assist you in determining how strong and how relevant the evidence is.

Put simply, you are trying to find out if it is worth looking at the study and the results, and whether the results are relevant to your practice.

- Critical appraisal tools help you develop a **consistent** approach to the critique of research and other information.

- They **only help** with the critical appraisal – they do not do the work for you! If you do not understand the methods by which the research has been undertaken, the tool will not help you. Therefore, you need to understand **what impacts on the quality and relevance** of each type of research you use so that you can appraise it. Some general reading about research methods will help with this.
- When you use a paper as evidence, it is important to **judge** its quality, not just report what the paper says.

Benefits and cautions when using an appraisal tool

The review process is complex and use of an appraisal tool will assist in the development of a systematic approach to this process and ensure that all papers are reviewed with equal rigour. Critical appraisal tools will guide you through questions you need to ask of each type of paper you have. Some tools ask questions that, if used simplistically, can result in the appraiser **simply reporting** what the paper says rather than forming a judgement. Anyone can report the findings of a paper – it takes skill to make a judgement as to the value of the results. This is where it is important that as an appraiser you have a good understanding of which factors influence quality in different types of research. There are many appraisal tools available online and in research textbooks and new ones are consistently being produced. For example, Downes et al. (2016) recently developed a tool for reviewing cross-sectional studies.

Before you opt for an appraisal tool, however, some researchers have cautioned that although widely available, few studies have addressed the rigour and usefulness of the tools themselves (see, for example, Katrak et al. 2004; Crowe and Sheppard 2011; Launey et al. 2016).

Starting with a general appraisal tool

Using a search engine (such as Google) will enable you to identify a good many of the available critical appraisal tools. You will also find examples in research or study skills textbooks and research or evidence-based practice journals.

For those of you new to critical appraisal, we recommend our **Six Questions for Critical Thinking** appraisal tool (Aveyard et al. 2015: 19). This tool has been developed for use with any piece of evidence and prompts the user to consider aspects of evidence-based practice we consider throughout this book.

Six Questions for Critical Thinking

Use the following **six questions** to help you analyse and appraise verbal or written information/evidence in practice and education (see guidance below)

1 **What** is it?	**Make notes here**
• What type of evidence is it? For example, is it a literature review, a research study, guidelines, personal opinion, a discussion paper, a website, or another type of evidence? • What are the findings/results or key points and are they relevant to what you want to know? *Why is this important?*	
2 **Where** did you find it? • Did you just 'come across' it? Who told you? Or did you access it through a systematic search using a professional database? *Why is this important?*	
3 **Who** wrote/said this? • Is it an individual representing their own viewpoint, or an individual/group representing an organization? • Are they experts on the topic? How do you know? *Why is this important?*	
4 **When** was it written/said? • Older key information may still be valid, but you need to check if there has been more recent work. *Why is this important?*	
5 **Why** was it written/said? • Who is the information aimed at – public, professionals, patient/client groups? • What is the aim of the information? • Could there be a hidden agenda? • Could there be any bias? How do you know? *Why is this important?*	

6 **How** do you know if it is of good quality? • How have the authors come to their conclusions? • Are the research methods used and/or line of reasoning logical, robust, and understandable? • Are there any flaws in the authors' arguments or approach? *Why is this important?*	
SO WHAT? • Is this the 'best available' evidence to inform your academic writing and/or practice? • Is this enough information or do you need to find more? • How will this now impact on your thinking and practice?	

What is it? It is very important that you can recognize the different types of information/evidence that you have. In general, well-conducted research is the strongest form of evidence. For all types of information/ evidence, you need to judge the quality of the arguments or evidence presented. It is also important to be able to summarize the findings.

Where did you find it? Whether you are doing an assignment or dissertation, or searching for evidence to inform practice, it is important to get the best available information/evidence. Evidence that you find as a result of a systematic search will be stronger than relying on the first information that comes to hand.

Who wrote/said this? It is important to identify whether the authors include their relevant qualifications and have the experience to write or speak authoritatively on the topic. For research, it is also particularly important that they have the necessary clinical, professional, and/or academic expertise to undertake the research.

When was it written/said? It is important to consider the date of information/publication. Older information will still be valid if it is considered 'key or seminal' (i.e. it is still widely referenced and used in more recent texts). However, you should check to determine whether there are newer theories or research that may be equally or more valid.

Why was it written/said? It is important to consider that information will be tailored differently to meet the different needs of different groups. You should also consider any agendas, conflicts or incentives (hidden or open).

How do you know if it is of good quality? This question incorporates all the questions above in addition to considering the overall quality or analysis of the information/evidence. Consider whether the arguments presented are robust and, if the information/evidence is research, whether the methods are appropriate to the study. Some understanding of research methods is useful here and a research methods textbook will help you develop your understanding.

The Six Questions for Critical Thinking is a generic tool that can be used on any evidence that you find and will help you to identify the type of evidence that you have.

Other general critical appraisal tools

Other general checklists are available to help you evaluate the evidence you come across and to think critically about arguments and evidence (see, for example, Melnyk 2016b). Further sources are given in Chapter 7 and in the Appendix, which details useful websites. Additionally, you will find appraisal tools in the appendix of many research textbooks and online. For example, Moule (2015) has developed a general appraisal tool that prompts the reader to consider the following areas (with sub-questions):

1 The purpose of the study
2 Research problem and research questions
3 Literature searches and review
4 Ethical issues
5 Sample selection
6 Research design and data collection
7 Results and analysis of findings
8 Conclusions, recommendations, and limitations
9 General points

Specific critical appraisal tools

If you need to use a more detailed tool, it is probably best to use a specific critical appraisal tool that is relevant to the type of research you are using.

If you have already had some experience of critical appraisal, you may wish to use a more specific critical appraisal tool that focuses on a specific research methodology. Appraisal tools that are specifically focused on a particular type of research paper will contain questions that are closely related to the study design in question, providing an appropriate structure for the review. Many critical appraisal tools have been developed for the review of specific types of research, and as such are **design specific,** for example, for the review of randomized controlled trials only.

There are many sources of critical appraisal tools, from specific professional groups and disciplines to academic and clinical institutions. It is worth searching to find one you like or is relevant (check the date and authors too). The following are a few examples; there are more in Chapter 7 and the Appendix.

Critical appraisal tools (sometimes known as CATs)

One of the most widely used sets of appraisal tools arises out of the **Critical Appraisal Skills Programme** (CASP International 2017). CASP has produced critical appraisal tools for use with many different types of research, including RCTs, systematic reviews, cohort and case control studies, and qualitative studies [available at: http://www.casp-uk.net/casp-international]

The Oxford-based **Centre for Evidence-Based Medicine** (CEBM) has different appraisal tools for systematic reviews, RCTs, diagnostic and prognosis studies, some of which are available in languages other than English [available at: http://www.cebm.net/critical-appraisal]

The **Joanna Briggs Institute** lists a substantial number of appraisal tools [available at: http://joannabriggs.org/research/critical-appraisal-tools.html]

For examples and to read more widely about appraisal, see http://www.students4bestevidence.net/category/appraising-research/

As a novice appraiser and at undergraduate level, you may initially consider the main questions in an appraisal tool, and only when you are more experienced or more widely read consider the additional more detailed questions. You will need access to a research textbook, glossary or dictionary to look up what you don't understand.

With all appraisal tools, when considering your answer to each question, you will need to evaluate the method – not just describe it.

We have found that many students have a tendency to describe the study rather than come to a conclusion about its quality. In order to help you evaluate, rather than just describe, the following are some prompt questions adapted from Sharp and Taylor (2012) to help you use two of the CASP appraisal tools – one for RCTs and one for qualitative research (see p. 158 and 165).

Key questions to ask when reviewing different types of evidence

We now discuss the **key questions** you should ask of the different types of evidence you are likely to encounter and provide some examples of critical appraisal tools you will find useful. Remember you can look at the specific tools and prompt questions if relevant. The different types of evidence are:

- Review articles and literature reviews
- Quantitative studies
- Qualitative studies
- Professional and clinical guidelines and policy
- Non-research information, for example, discussion and opinion or anecdotal evidence
- Websites.

Key questions to ask of review articles and literature reviews

We have discussed the value of systematic reviews and good quality literature reviews in detail throughout this book. We suggest the following questions should be asked to determine if the review is of good quality.

Has the review been undertaken systematically?

When evaluating review articles, you should be able to determine whether the review was undertaken in an explicit systematic way or whether a more haphazard and random approach has been used. A review incorporating a systematic approach will present stronger evidence than a review that does not.

Are the researchers explicit about the methods?

You should check if the authors have said clearly how they undertook the review, what keywords or terms they used, over what period, how they decided what to include, etc. The amount of detail given to the search, critiquing and bringing together the evidence, will differ with each literature review. You should scrutinize the methods used to conduct the review.

Do the researchers demonstrate that they did everything in their power to ensure their approach was as systematic as possible? If the review is described as a **Cochrane** or **Campbell Collaboration review**, you can be fairly confident that it was undertaken systematically. Resources are available that guide such reviews to ensure consistency [see http://training.cochrane.org/handbook or https://campbellcollaboration.org/research-resources/writing-a-campbell-systematic-review.html].

Example

A Cochrane-style systematic review aims to uncover **all literature** on the topic in question. It will involve a team of researchers, who work together with explicit criteria in the selection and critical analysis of the literature.

A less detailed review is likely to be carried out by a single researcher with fewer resources for collaboration in these aspects. A less detailed review will acknowledge that the search is unlikely to be exhaustive but is likely to **identify the databases used**.

Try and find a systematic review relating to your profession using a database or the Cochrane Library [http://www.cochranelibrary.com/] or Campbell Collaboration [https://www.campbellcollaboration.org/library.html].

Example of a critical appraisal tool for review articles

One of the critical appraisal tools for the appraisal of a systematic review is the CASP tool for systematic reviews [available at: http://www.casp-uk.net/casp-international].

Key questions to ask of quantitative studies

In Chapter 4, we describe two main approaches to quantitative studies – experimental and non-experimental.

Using a database, try to find a quantitative study relating to your profession.

We now outline the key questions you need to ask of quantitative research.

What method was selected to undertake the research?

Most papers will provide a short summary of the research process undertaken and from this you will be able to identify how the study was conducted. Make sure you understand the method. Guidelines to enhance good practice in research are available at the Equator network [http://www.equator-network.org/]. Equator publish standards or guidelines for researchers to adhere to, including the **CONSORT** Statement to guide those undertaking randomized controlled trials. It comprises a 25-item checklist to focus on reporting how the trial was designed, analysed, and interpreted; the flow diagram displays the progress of all participants through the trial.

What was the sample size?

The sample size refers to the number of participants in the study. The authors of quantitative research papers should demonstrate how they determined the sample size for the research in question. This should be clearly documented in the paper and is often referred to as a **power calculation**.

A power calculation is a statistical test undertaken when designing a research study in order to estimate if the sample is large enough for the findings to be considered reliable.

Example

The findings of a small study are likely to be less reliable than those of a larger study, as they may be due to chance variations. With a larger sample, the findings are less likely to be due to chance.

Has an appropriate sample been obtained?

You need to ask yourself, **who was selected to participate** in the study? Quantitative research sometimes uses **random sampling**, which means that the sample was chosen at random from the overall population. When you are reviewing a quantitative study, be aware of the sampling strategy and be able to comment on the reasons as to why this approach has been adopted. Consider whether a random or non-random sample was used and whether this was appropriate. Remember that, as explained in Chapter 4, **randomization** or **random allocation** is different from random sampling.

How were the data collected?

The data collection method should be **appropriate** for the study design. Quantitative research uses a wide range of data collection methods that are appropriate for objective measurement such as survey/question-naires, symptom ratings, objective physiological tests, observation, and rates of occurrence (incidence). *Note how researchers say the data were collected (not was collected).*

How were the data analysed?

Quantitative data are usually analysed statistically and you should expect to find reference to the statistical tests used in the paper in order to make sense of the data. There should be numerical presentation of the data and discussion of these findings. You might expect to see terms such as **confidence intervals** and **statistical significance** including *p*-value discussed. There will probably be a section entitled **main findings/ results**. You should consider if the data analysis is **objective**.

Resources for reviewing RCTs

The CASP (2017) critical appraisal tool for RCTs is available online. The following supplementary prompt questions were developed from Sharp and Taylor (2012):

Additional prompt questions to help you evaluate rather than simply report. You should answer 'yes', 'no' or 'cannot tell' and be able to provide reasons.

1 *Did the trial address a clearly focused issue?*

   ☐ Is the question or aim clearly stated and rationale given? Tip: a question should have a question mark (?) at the end of it.

   ☐ Why is it important to have a clearly focused question or stated aim?

   ☐ Does it contain all the elements of a PICOT question?

2 *Was the assignment of patients to treatments randomized?*

☐ How well were participants allocated to different groups?

☐ Was the randomization done in an objective way?

3 *Were all of the participants who entered the trial properly accounted for at its conclusion?*

☐ Did any participants who started in the study fail to complete? Tip: did more people drop out in the intervention group than the control group? Why might this matter?

☐ Why is 'loss to follow up' important for this study's findings?

☐ Was intention-to-treat analysis undertaken and why is it important?

4 *Were the participants, health workers, and study personnel 'blind' to treatments?*

☐ Was double or single blinding possible and, if so, was it achieved? Tip: consider the patients/clients, researchers, and professional staff where relevant.

☐ Why is it important and what are the implications of the blinding approach?

5 *Were the groups similar at the start of the trial?*

☐ Were the groups matched in terms of age, sex, location, etc.? Was stratified randomization used?

☐ Can you notice any potential unreported differences between the two groups?

☐ Is this important for this study and why?

6 *Aside from the experimental intervention, were the groups treated equally?*

☐ Were there or could there be any differences (variables) that might have influenced the group besides the intervention and would it make any difference to the results of this study? Tip: consider how the intervention was delivered/administered (were different staff or equipment involved?).

7 *How large was the treatment effect?*

☐ Were the measurable outcomes thoroughly reported (consider rigour and if any results are missing)?

☐ What was the difference in outcome between the control and experimental group, i.e. what were the findings/results?

☐ Was a power calculation conducted? How might the sample size impact on the results of *this* study? (Note: you can discuss the statistics in the next question.)

8 *How precise was the estimate of the treatment effect?*

☐ Are there any inconsistencies (or errors) between the statistics presented and the discussion or conclusions drawn?
☐ Are the results statistically significant? What does this mean?
☐ Did the authors use *p*-values and confidence intervals/limits? Why is this useful?

9 *Can the results be applied to the local population?*

☐ Are the participants similar to your own?
Tip: consider culture, gender, setting, severity of problem/ condition, etc.
☐ Do any differences matter? If so, why? (Don't make the assumptions that research carried out in another country is not relevant.)
☐ How do the findings relate to what currently happens in your setting? Might you consider changing practice as a result of this study?

10 *Were all clinically important outcomes considered?*

☐ What did the authors not consider that might have influenced the results?
☐ Overall, is this study of good enough quality to be useful?
☐ Given all the points you have made above, how generalizable are the results?
☐ Is further research needed?

11 *Are the benefits worth the harms and costs?*

☐ Is the intervention worth adopting in practice and policy?
☐ Is it too expensive to adopt? Consider staff, training, and equipment.
☐ Are the side effects/or any harm worth it?

Resources when reviewing cohort studies and case control studies

A CASP critical appraisal tool for cohort studies and case control studies is available on their website [http://www.casp-uk.net/casp-international]. The Joanna Briggs Institute also has tools for cohort studies and case control studies [http://joannabriggs.org/research/critical-appraisal-tools.html].

Resources when reviewing surveys/questionnaires

On one level, surveys and questionnaires are easy to critique as we are all familiar with the method of research. It is unlikely that anyone reading this book has not completed a questionnaire or survey at some point and also formed an opinion as to the relevance of the questionnaire, which may have ended up in the bin rather than back in the researcher's office! The few appraisal tools for questionnaires/surveys have often been poorly devised. CASP and CEBM do not offer appraisal tools for questionnaires.

Think of a time you found a questionnaire hard to answer or when the meaning of the questions was unclear.

We have simplified Greenhalgh's (2014) detailed checklist below to provide you with some good questions to ask when reviewing questionnaires and surveys:

1 Is a questionnaire the best way to find out the information?
2 Is there already a validated questionnaire available and did the authors use it? If not, why not?
3 Have the authors discussed the reliability and validity of the questionnaire?
4 Was the questionnaire well presented, well structured, and phrased suitably for the health literacy of the participants?
5 Were clear instructions and explanations given?
6 Was a pilot study of the questionnaire carried out and amended if need be?
7 Was the sample size large enough and did it represent the population group adequately?
8 Was the questionnaire distributed and administered in an appropriate way (for example, by post, digitally – apps, e-surveys, email – or telephone) and was it self-administered or researcher-assisted?
9 Were issues such as literacy levels, different languages, etc. considered? Was the response rate high? If not (< 70%), have the researchers discussed any potential differences between those who responded and those who didn't and the impact on the results?
10 Was the data analysis appropriate and did it relate to the question/hypothesis?
11 What were the results? Were they statistically significant and all results including negative and insignificant ones reported?
12 If there were qualitative responses, have they been reported and interpreted adequately and have qualitative data (e.g. free text responses) been adequately and reasonably presented? Were 'quotes' used carefully to represent the findings?
13 What were the results and have the researchers realistically presented a link between the data presented and their conclusions?

An additional appraisal tool devised by Roever (2015) is available at: https://www.omicsonline.org/open-access/critical-appraisal-of-a-questionnaire-study-ebmp-1000e110.php?aid=70356

The next time you find a questionnaire, or are asked to complete one, try and critically appraise it using some of the principles outlined above.

Key questions to ask of qualitative studies

There has been much discussion in recent years concerning the ways in which qualitative research is evaluated and this debate is ongoing.

This is because there is often no set approach or standard for carrying out qualitative research and methods are being developed all the time (Noble and Smith 2015), and so it can be difficult to evaluate.

Most qualitative researchers argue that it is not possible to assess qualitative research in the same way as quantitative research. For this reason, researchers such as Lincoln and Guba (1985) and Noble and Smith (2015) argue that the **following terms are more appropriate** for assessing the quality of a qualitative study:

- **Credibility** – do the findings ring true from the approach taken? Are they well presented and meaningful?
- **Transferability/applicability** – can the results be transferred to different settings/groups?
- **Dependability** – can you rely on the results as they are presented?
- **Confirmability** – could the study be repeated?

Try to identify a qualitative research study by accessing a database and looking at the titles and abstracts.

Remember that critical appraisal of qualitative research is complex. When reviewing qualitative research, you need to be familiar with the approaches to qualitative study that were used in the papers you have identified.

The key questions of qualitative research you need to ask are:

Was a qualitative method appropriate?

Consider whether a qualitative method was appropriate for the study and specifically whether the use of words and an in-depth exploration was the best way to collect data for the study.

Who was the sample?

You would expect to see purposive, theoretical, convenience or snowball sampling. Do the researchers give a clear rationale for their sampling approach? What types of participant make up the purposive sample and are they the most relevant?

How large was the sample?

You would expect the sample size to be large enough to achieve sufficient information-rich cases for in-depth data analysis (called data saturation), but not so large that the amount of data obtained becomes unmanageable. Has the way in which the sample size was arrived at been clearly explained?

How were the data collected?

It is important that the researchers justify the approach they have taken to the data collection process and can demonstrate that the process was undertaken systematically and rigorously. The way of collecting the data should also be appropriate to the method and research question. Most researchers agree that in-depth **interviews and focus groups** should be tape-recorded so that the interviews can be **transcribed** (an exact word-for-word account of what was said). However, some researchers argue that this is time-consuming and that the time could be better used by undertaking additional interviews and hence collecting considerably more data. Qualitative questionnaires/surveys are sometimes used and the response population would need to be considered here too.

Is a rationale given for the data collection approach?

Is the reason for **interviews, focus groups or qualitative question-naires** (and, more recently, data collected via social media) clearly stated?

Focus groups are a form of group interview and may be selected over in-depth interviews when dialogue **between research participants** is considered beneficial. If the research topic is unfamiliar to those involved and participants may not have developed their thoughts in relation to the topic under study, focus groups can be useful as a data collection method because the ideas expressed by one participant may trigger a response in another participant. Ask yourself whether the researchers have considered the disadvantages (limitations) of the approaches used.

Example

If a topic is particularly sensitive, participants may be reluctant to express their thoughts in a focus group, so in-depth interviews may be more appropriate.

Questionnaires can be used for the collection of **qualitative data**. While it is possible to collect qualitative data through open-ended questions on a questionnaire schedule, such data are unlikely to be as in depth as data collected through one-to-one interaction.

Social media is an emerging area for research and McKee (2013) notes that content from Twitter, Facebook, etc. is being seen as a source of data for surveillance or monitoring, for example, the concerns or commentary of the public. She outlines that there are ethical issues to consider in accessing this type of data, as the boundary between what is public and private is blurred.

Observational data may be used in both quantitative and qualitative studies if researchers want to see what people actually do rather than what they say they do. Data collected through **observation** is especially useful for this. If the observed activity is counted, it would be a quantitative approach, and if described and interpreted, it would be a qualitative approach. For example, the number of infection control practices undertaken by each practitioner could be counted numerically, or the nature of the interaction between practitioner and patient could be observed using qualitative approaches. Researchers need to consider the **Hawthorne effect**, which refers to the tendency of people who are observed to behave differently (usually better) than they would usually (McCambridge et al. 2014).

Who collected the data?

Is the interviewer **trained and skilled** in asking questions that probe the experience of the participant and is the aim clearly stated in order to generate rich data through one-to-one dialogue? Did more than one interviewer carry out the interviews and if so what might be the impact? Did they discuss their relationship with the participants openly?

How were the data analysed?

Word restrictions impose limitations on the detail that can be given in any journal paper, but there should be evidence of a considered approach to data analysis. Did more than one person try and independently code the data or identify the themes? Did they use direct quotes from the participants to represent the themes?

Has a computer package been used to analyse the data?

This in itself does not ensure rigour in the analysis process, but you might expect to see some acknowledgement of the possibilities for data analysis using different methods. It is possible to demonstrate rigour in data analysis without the use of computer packages.

Is there justification as to how much data was collected?

The researchers should seek to justify how many interviews or focus groups or other forms of qualitative data they collected. Was data saturation achieved? Data saturation means that at the end of the analysis period, the continuing data analysis does not identify additional new themes from the data, but instead the data analysed merely add to the existing themes that have emerged from previous data analysis.

Resources when reviewing qualitative studies

There is a CASP tool for qualitative research [see http://www.casp-uk.net/casp-international]. See also the prompt questions offered below adapted from (Sharp and Taylor 2012).

Additional prompt questions to help you evaluate rather than simply report using the CASP (2017) qualitative tool

1 *Was there a clear statement of the aims of the research?*

☐   Did the authors ask clearly focused questions, or state an aim? Why is this important?

☐   Can you relate it to qualitative PICOT (see Stillwell et al. 2010)? Tip: a question should have a question mark (?) at the end of it.

2 *Is a qualitative methodology appropriate?*

☐   How does this study reflect the broad key characteristics of qualitative research?

☐   Given the aim/question of *this* study, why is qualitative research more appropriate than quantitative research?

3 *Was the research design appropriate to address the aims of the research?*

☐   How well have the researchers designed this study? Have they used a particular qualitative approach (e.g. phenomenology, action research, ethnography)? Did they justify their approach adequately?

☐   What are the advantages/limitations of this study's design compared with those of another design they might have considered? Do the advantages of their chosen design outweigh the limitations in order to achieve their research aims? Why?

4 *Was the recruitment strategy appropriate to the aims of the research?*

☐   How were people recruited? What sampling approach (convenience, purposive, snowballing) was used? Did any potential participants refuse and were reasons why discussed?

☐   How did the researchers define and justify the strategy that they used? Did the population selected provide the type of knowledge sought by the study?

☐   What are the advantages/disadvantages of this strategy for this study's aims?

☐   Is there anything that the researchers overlooked?

☐   What are the implications of this for the findings of *this* study?

5 *Were the data collected in a way that addressed the research issues?*

☐   How and where were the data collected (structured, unstructured, semi-structured interviews, focus groups, etc.)? How well has it been described and justified by the researchers?

☐   Why was this method of data collection particularly useful for this study's aims? Were alternatives considered?

☐   Have the researchers considered and reached data saturation?

☐   Is there anything that the researchers overlooked (impact of setting, skill of the researchers)?

☐   What are the implications of this for *this* study's findings?

6 *Has the relationship between researcher and participants been adequately considered?*

☐   What was the relationship? Did the researchers acknowledge the potential impact (positive or negative)?

☐ Was reflexivity discussed? What is this? What purpose does it serve? Did this study demonstrate reflexivity (e.g. diaries, logs, discussion)?

☐ How did the researchers enable/restrict the participants' ability to talk about their experiences on this topic?

☐ What might they have overlooked?

☐ What are the implications for *this* study's findings?

7 **Have ethical issues been taken into account?**

☐ What ethical issues/principles did they consider?

☐ Did they submit to an ethical approval committee?

☐ Are there any ethical issues that the researchers overlooked?

☐ What are the implications for the findings of *this* study?

8 **Was the data analysis sufficiently rigorous?**

☐ Did the researchers explain thoroughly how they analysed the data, including identifying any themes?
Tip: Consider credibility, dependability, and trustworthiness.

☐ Did they use more than one person to identify/confirm the themes?

☐ Did they use respondent validation (member checking)? What is this? How necessary is it for their research design?

☐ Is there anything that the researchers overlooked – were there any contradictions?

☐ What are the implications for the findings of *this* study?

9 **Is there a clear statement of findings?**

☐ What are the findings? How do the themes and sub-themes emerge from the data?

☐ Do the findings clearly and accurately emerge from the data?

10 **How valuable is the research?**

☐ Think about the purpose of qualitative research findings (insight, understanding). Evaluate how useful the study's findings are for practice in the light of the quality of the study.

We have simplified Greenhalgh's (2014) checklist for qualitative research below:

1 Are the context and importance of the problem clearly stated in the form of a question? *(See information on PICOT questions in Chapter 5.)*

2 Was the qualitative approach appropriate?

3 How were the place for the research and the participants chosen? *(See discussion on sample selection and size in qualitative research below.)*

4 What was the researcher's perspective/involvement, and has this been taken into account and described? *(Look up reflexive/reflexivity.)*
5 Has the researcher described the data collection methods in detail?
6 How did they analyse the data to ensure that it was credible and of a high standard?
7 Are the results credible and, if so, are they relevant and applicable to practice?
8 Are the conclusions drawn clearly from the results?
9 Are the findings of the study transferable to other settings? *(See definition above.)*

Key questions to ask of mixed methods research

Mixed methods research focuses on both numeric and narrative data and analysis and is increasingly used to combine the benefits of both methods and hence increase applicability to the population (Graff 2016). You may want to use a combination of different appraisal tools for the mixed methods used in the research. The National Collaborating Centre for Methods and Tools (NCCMT 2015) has developed the Mixed Methods Appraisal Tool (MMAT) [available at: http://www.nccmt.ca/resources/search/232]. Souto et al. (2015) have evaluated the usefulness of the tool and concluded that MMAT is an efficient tool, but its reliability needs some improvement. The authors concluded that the appraisal of the quality of studies with diverse designs remains challenging.

Considering ethical issues in research

For all research involving participants, ethical principles and guidance need to be considered as part of critical appraisal. You should look for ethical committee approval, signs of coercion (particularly with vulnerable people, respecting confidentiality, anonymity, and human dignity). Glasper (2015: 38) provides a detailed flow chart that shows how ethics need to be considered at all stages of the research process: planning, application to ethics committee, data collection and dissemination. Look at the World Medical Association publication, the 'Declaration of Helsinki: ethical principles for medical research involving human subjects' (2013), and Beauchamp and Childress's (2013) widely used ethical principles are below:

- Autonomy – this applies to individuals and organizations.
- Beneficence (do good) – this is considered a core value in health and social care.

- Non-maleficence (do no harm) – this can be linked to beneficence, i.e. if we do good, we do no harm.
- Justice – social benefits, resources, and burdens are distributed with integrity.

Key questions to ask of professional and clinical guidance and policy

As with any publication, professional and clinical guidance and policy vary in quality and should be appraised. As we have already stated, ideally these guidelines and policy documents should be **based on the best available evidence**. However, it is still up to you to ensure that the advice given in the protocol is up to date and useful. Indeed, this should be the first question you ask of the guidelines or policy. Make a decision that, from now on, you will ask yourself questions about the validity of the guidelines or policies you have to work with, rather than just accepting this at face value. There is a growing literature on the evaluation, appraisal, and updating of clinical practice guidelines (e.g. Kredo et al. 2016; Siering et al. 2013). Consider what you would do, as an accountable practitioner, if clinical and professional guidelines or policy within your workplace were not up to date or evidence-based.

> The Agree Collaboration offers guidance on the development of guidelines and also a **critical appraisal tool for assessing the quality of guidelines and policy** [the AGREE 11 tool is available at: http://www.agreetrust.org/].
>
> The National Institute of Health and Care Excellence (NICE) has a clinical practice guidelines manual (2014) [available at: https://www.nice.org.uk/process/pmg20/chapter/introduction-and-overview].

We have simplified Greenhalgh's (2014) checklist for clinical or professional guidelines below:

1 Was there any conflict of interest in the preparation and publication?
2 Are the guidelines appropriate to your topic, and do they identify the expected outcomes in terms of health and/or cost?
3 Was someone who has expertise in bringing together evidence (meta-analysis) involved?
4 Are the conclusions based on scrutiny of all the available and relevant data?

5 Do they address controversial areas such as funding and inequalities?
6 Are they valid and reliable?
7 Are they detailed, flexible, and relevant to practice?
8 Are they acceptable to, affordable by, and realistic for patients/clients to adopt?
9 Do they state how they can be shared, implemented, reviewed, and evaluated?

 Find out where professional and clinical guidelines specifically relevant to your practice might be published.

Key questions to ask of discussion/opinion papers

When you come across non-research-based evidence, it is important that you recognize this and are equipped to assess its usefulness. Try using our **Six Questions to Trigger Critical Thinking** (Aveyard et al. 2015) to help you consider the quality and purpose of what you are reading.

McArthur et al. (2015: 3) offer a critical appraisal tool for text and opinion that is available on The Joanna Briggs Institute website [see http:// joannabriggs.org/research/critical-appraisal-tools.html]:

1. Is the source of the opinion clearly identified?

2. Does the source of opinion have standing in the field of expertise?

3. Are the interests of the relevant population the central focus of the opinion?

4. Is the stated position the result of an analytical process, and is there logic in the opinion expressed?

5. Is there reference to the extant literature?

6. Is any incongruence with the literature/sources logically defended?

Another approach to reviewing a paper is to assess the quality of the arguments presented (relating to question 4 above). Thouless and Thouless (1953) first advocated this approach when discussing the use of logic in a constructed argument presented in a discussion paper. They articulate 38 **dishonest tricks** commonly used in an argument or written discussion. These include:

• Using emotionally charged words
• Making conclusive statements using words such as 'all' when 'some' would be more appropriate or 'never' when 'rarely' would be more appropriate

- Using selected instances or examples
- Misrepresentation of opposing arguments
- Not mentioning counter-arguments.

Does the evidence on which the arguments are founded bear scrutiny?

If the arguments are well constructed and defensible, then greater weight can be given to them than others that are less well prepared and constructed. You should question the use of language, the acknowledgement of alternative approaches or lines of argument, forced analogy, and false credentials. Cottrell (2017) offers useful ideas on reviewing arguments in written work. It is important to remember that the expert opinion of a well-known figure in the area might be found to contradict established findings from empirical research.

Can you identify three things you might now do differently when reading professional literature?

Key questions to ask of websites

Should I believe all information contained on websites?

The answer is, of course, NO! It is true that the Internet contains a wealth of information that is useful to health and social care practitioners and our patients/clients. However, as we have seen, there is also a wealth of poor quality and misleading information. Many websites are unregulated, on which it is possible for anybody to publish anything they like. You must, therefore, be critical of any website you encounter. We recommend using our **Six Questions to Trigger Critical Thinking** (Aveyard et al. 2015) to get you started.

- The web contains many hundreds of millions of pages, from rigorous research to trivia and misinformation.
- Before making use of information found on the web in your academic work, you need to make sure it is of high quality.
- You should also remember that if you use information from the web in your academic work, then, just like printed sources, those web pages must be cited in the reference list of your thesis, paper, etc. (see if your organization or university has a guide to referencing).

- Kitchens et al. (2014) found that web searches for terms related to preventive health and social health issues tend to produce lower quality results than terms related to diagnosis and treatment of physical disease or injury.

Evaluating websites

Evaluating the quality of web resources

When evaluating the quality of web resources, consider the following **ABC** (adapted from Howe 2001, revised 2010): **A**ccuracy, **A**uthority, **B**ias, **B**readth and depth, **C**omparison, **C**urrency [see http://www.walthowe.com/navnet/quality.html].

Accuracy – finding 'facts' or figures quoted on the web is not an automatic guarantee that the information is accurate. Can you check the information against other sources? Does it fit with what you already know? Do the authors of the page tell you where they got the information from?

Authority – who is providing the information, and what evidence do you have that they know what they are talking about? It is not always easy to see immediately where a particular web page comes from, and an impressive-looking, flashy web page is not necessarily a guarantee of good quality information! If you have found the page via a link or a search engine, look for a 'Home', 'Front Page' or similar icon, and follow it to try to see whether the page authors are well-known experts, and whether they provide a mission statement, 'real-world' postal address and phone number, or a bibliography of their other articles, reports or books.

Bias – as with any source of information, it is possible for a web page to appear objective, but in fact be promoting a particular standpoint. Be critical. For example, if you have found information on a particular drug, are the writers of this web page from the company that makes the drug, from a campaign group trying to get the drug banned or from an independent research institute?

Breadth and depth of information – how detailed is the information? What evidence is given to support it? Does it cover all relevant areas of the subject? Does the web page link to further relevant sources of information?

Comparison with other sources – to provide confidence in the information you find, compare it with other sources of information on the subject: published statistics, journal articles, textbooks or other websites.

Currency – it is easy to assume that information on the web must be very current (up to date), whereas in fact many pages have not been updated for years. How current does your information need to be? Does the page say when it was last updated? (If not, try checking the Properties or Page Info option in your web browser and see if a date is given.) Do all the links to other sites still work? Remember, even if the page has been updated recently, all the information may not have been checked.

A useful guide to **evaluating web sources** is available from Oxford Brookes University Library [see http://www.brookes.ac.uk/library/webeval.html] that includes:

- What is being said?
- Who is saying it?
- Where are they from?
- Why are they saying it?
- When does this information date from?

Also, remember that there are a range of pre-evaluated 'subject gateways' available on the web, where experts have searched the web for high-quality, reliable information. These will be explored in detail in the next chapter (see also the Appendix).

Incorporating critical appraisal into your academic writing and in practice

So far in this chapter, we have considered ways of making sense of research and non-research evidence you may encounter. Overall, the purpose of critical appraisal is to enable you to make sense of the evidence you come across. It takes you from a position of '*do not believe everything you read*' to one of where you have the skills to assess and evaluate what you read so that you can determine the strengths and weaknesses of the evidence you encounter. It is important to remember that you need to critically appraise – make sense of – all the evidence you read, whether you are using that evidence in your practice or in your academic writing. However, when you are using evidence in your academic work, it is useful to be mindful of the following points:

- Make sure that it is clear that you have read, understood the relevance and quality of evidence you are using.

- Consider if you have only one 'piece of the jigsaw puzzle' and if you need to find more evidence to get the whole picture and present the evidence in practice or in your writing.
- Remember to provide information about the **type of evidence** you are using. If it is a research study, say so; if it is a discussion article, state this.
- Resist the temptation to paraphrase or quote without evaluative comment. Make sure you give the context of the evidence you use.
- Try not to 'cherry-pick' the evidence to support what you want to say; instead, search your topic with an 'open mind' and you may find (and be able to use) something you didn't know about beforehand.
- If you find one viewpoint or piece of evidence, sometimes it is worth searching for the contrary view so that you have the different sides of an argument, enabling you to compare and contrast.
- Don't forget that if you have evaluated the research as poor quality, you should not give much weight to the results.

Example of how to show the context and value of the information source

We suggest that you avoid writing: *'Jones (2015) argues that university students prefer lectures to tutorials'* (we do not know who Jones is or how Jones has reached this conclusion).

We suggest instead that you write: *'In a small questionnaire study, Jones (2015) found that 70% of students preferred lectures to tutorials.'*

Or: *'Jones (2015) argues that from his own experience as a student in London, there was strong feeling among his peer group that lectures were preferable to tutorials.'*

As can be seen in the example above, it is important to distinguish between a research study based on evidence, and if so what type of evidence, or merely an opinion. This is relevant whether you are debating the use of evidence in practice or in academic writing.

 As a general rule, avoid writing a statement and only giving the author's name, such as 'Jones (2015) says', as the reader is completely unaware of the context of Jones's work.

In summary

Once you have found your evidence, it is vital that you are able to look at it objectively and then work out first what it is, and, second, whether it helps you to address what you need to find out. The purpose of critical appraisal is to determine the relevance, strengths, and limitations of the information collected so that you can determine how helpful the evidence is in answering your question. A study might be well carried out but not very relevant to your research question. Alternatively, a study might be very relevant to your research question but not well designed or implemented. Furthermore, discussion and expert opinion and web-based sources might add interesting insight to your argument, but the quality of this information also needs to be assessed.

Key points

1 The first thing to do is identify whether you have a research paper or some other type of evidence.
2 You need to read and re-read any papers before you can begin to critically appraise.
3 Critical appraisal is a necessary process in determining the relevance and quality of the published information related to your research question.
4 You need to distinguish between papers that report empirical findings and those that present discussion or expert opinion only.
5 You are advised to use one of the many critical appraisal tools that are available to structure your critical appraisal.

Quiz questions

1 Why can we not accept everything we read in professional journals?
2 Why is peer review not perfect?
3 What are the advantages of using a critical appraisal tool to appraise research papers?

7 How to implement evidence-based practice

- *The challenge of getting more evidence into practice*
- *Individual motivation, skills, and competencies for evidence-based practice*
- *Organizational culture*
- *Finding solutions to the problems of implementing evidence-based practice*
- *Challenging our own practice and that of others*
- *The future of evidence-based practice*
- *In summary*
- *Key points*
- *Quiz questions*

In this chapter, we will:

- Give an overview of the context and reality of evidence-based practice, including the barriers to evidence implementation
- Explore motivational factors – both individual and organizational – and some of the roles that may contribute to the implementation of evidence
- Identify the skills needed by the evidence-based practitioner and how they can develop them further
- Offer a wider range of general and specific strategies and resources to help with accessing and using evidence in the reality of practice environments

- Consider ways that we can be constructively critical of our own and others' practice
- Recognize where further research is needed in evaluating the impact of EBP approaches.

The challenge of getting more evidence into practice

In the previous chapters of this book, we have emphasized how and why evidence-based practice has become so important. We have an ever-increasing supply of information that we need to make sense of, and increasingly well-informed or 'expert' patients to whom we are accountable and have a duty to provide safe and effective evidence-based care. In addition, we have a changing workforce – both nationally and internationally there are shortages of health and social care professionals together with changes to skill mix. This often means that registered practitioners are taking on wider leadership roles and are responsible for delegating evidence-based practice interventions and therapies to support workers. Increasingly, this means they have to justify reasons and decisions to others.

Throughout this book, we have outlined the steps you need to take when you define an area for exploration, and start to search for and evaluate the evidence you find. In a way, that's the easy bit. It's certainly the logical part. The relevance of evidence-based practice for safe and effective practice is clear to see. We would all prefer to be cared for by a practitioner who is up to date and accountable rather than a practitioner who is reliant on unreliable sources. Even searching for and evaluating the evidence is fairly straightforward once you have worked out how to do it.

Putting the evidence into practice and evaluating its effectiveness is what really matters. And here is the conundrum: knowing the value of evidence-based practice is not enough – you also need to implement an evidence-based approach in your practice. Melnyk et al. (2014: 5) stated:

> . . . although it is widely known that evidence-based practice (EBP) improves healthcare quality, reliability, and patient outcomes as well as reduces variations in care and costs, it is still not the standard of care delivered by practicing clinicians across the globe.

Rather alarmingly, Greenhalgh (2014) claims that **a lot** of avoidable suffering is caused by not implementing evidence-based practice. She warns that although there are strategies to improve the time it takes to get evidence into practice, there are no 'quick fixes'. It seems that the introduction of evidence-based practice is not as widespread as we would like to believe. Harvey and Kitson (2015a) note that the translation of research evidence into both policy and practice is an ongoing challenge in health systems worldwide. They add that changing the behaviour of individuals, teams, organizations, and systems is complex and conclude that effective strategies need to be individually tailored and multi-faceted. Any database search will readily find a plethora of both national and international literature about implementation and utilization of evidence within the health and social care professions. In an overview of systematic reviews, Squires et al. (2014) concluded that even the evidence about how to do this is inconclusive. Harvey and Kitson argue for a wider range of research methodologies for evaluating the context-dependent nature of getting research into practice.

Williams et al. (2015) note how different terms are used to discuss the concept of getting evidence into practice. Terms such as research utilization, uptake, and integration are described in the literature. Albrecht et al. (2016) describe **knowledge transfer** as a strategy to enhance the uptake of research findings, while the Centre for Reviews and Dissemination (CRD) describes **knowledge translation** as a process used to raise awareness and improve the impact of research findings [see https://www.york.ac.uk/crd/research/knowledge-transfer/]. Importantly, they add that evidence should be presented in a way that is accessible to different professional groups.

 The hardest part of evidence-based practice seems to be overcoming barriers, motivating individuals *and* organizations *to adopt an* evidence practice culture, *putting this* evidence into practice *and* evaluating its effectiveness.

Indeed, dissemination, implementation, and evaluation are part of evidence-based practice and once we know about the evidence, we need to use it and evaluate its use in practice. In presenting their seven steps to evidence-based practice, Melnyk and colleagues (2010) state that evaluation and dissemination of evidence are key to getting evidence into practice.

Why is it difficult to put evidence-based practice into practice?

Many researchers have found that practitioners have a willingness and enthusiasm to provide quality care and put evidence into practice (Friesen-Storms et al. 2014; Llasus et al. 2014; Leach et al. 2016). However, Gray et al. (2014) found that many clinicians favour experience and professional judgement over research evidence, which might reflect a lack of knowledge and understanding of evidence-based practice.

Despite this willingness, the challenge of getting evidence into practice is clear and has been the focus of much research in recent years. Gray et al. (2015), Mallion and Brooke (2016), Friesen-Storms et al. (2014), Heydari et al. (2014), Kajermo et al. (2010), Llasus et al. (2014), and Dogherty et al. (2013) have all come to similar conclusions about why it is difficult to put evidence into practice. These barriers are summarized by the Evidence-Based Practice Attitude and Utilization Survey (EBASE) (Leach and Gillham 2008). In part E, 13 barriers to the implementation of evidence are identified:

1 Lack of time
2 Lack of resources
3 Lack of clinical evidence in nursing
4 Inadequate skills for locating research
5 Inadequate skills for interpreting research
6 Inadequate skills to critically appraise/evaluate the literature
7 Inadequate skills to apply research findings to clinical practice
8 Lack of incentive to participate in evidence-based practice
9 Lack of interest in evidence-based practice
10 Lack of relevance to nursing practice
11 Lack of colleague support for evidence-based practice
12 Lack of industry support for evidence-based practice
13 Patient preference for treatment.

Many subsequent research projects (for example, Leach et al. 2016) undertaken in a wide variety of health and social care professions, have utilized the EBASE survey or another tool, all of which can be readily identified via a database search.

Jun et al. (2016) carried out an integrated review into barriers and facilitators of nurses' use of clinical practice guidelines. Attitudes, perceptions, and knowledge were identified as the internal barriers, while format and usability of clinical practice guidelines, resources, leadership, and organizational culture were considered external barriers and facilitators. Jun et al. (2016) assert that nurses are the gatekeepers of patient care and major players in the healthcare system. Therefore, nurses must play an active role in the development, implementation, and updating of clinical practice guidelines to ensure high-quality care to all patients.

In order to explore these barriers further, Williams et al. (2015) have used the BARRIERS Scale with an international group of occupational therapists. This 19-item version of the BARRIERS Scale appears to be applicable in cross-cultural settings and is regarded as a robust, valid, and reliable measure, although further evaluation in other professional groups is recommended (for a systematic review and further detail of the scale, see Kajermo et al. 2010). Williams et al. (2015) found both individual and organizational factors are involved, emphasizing the complex nature of implementing evidence-based practice. In the next section, we consider what we can do both at an individual and an organizational level to reduce the barriers to an evidence-based approach in professional practice.

 Once you have finished reading this chapter, try adopting the ideas presented here to help you overcome some of these barriers.

Individual motivation, skills, and competencies for evidence-based practice

The role of the individual is clearly important for pulling down these barriers. The individual practitioner needs to have certain motivations, knowledge, skills, and competencies in order to adopt evidence-based practices. These, together with resources, infrastructure, and leadership, are most likely to result in the best outcomes for our patients/clients.

As we identified in Chapter 1, the first step to getting evidence into practice is described as 'igniting a spirit of enquiry' (Melnyk et al. 2009). This implies that there is a spark or trigger that gets us to start thinking and questioning what we do. This fits well with educational strategies encouraging critical thinking, curiosity, and a sceptical approach to information (Aveyard et al. 2015).

Readiness or motivation

A spirit of enquiry requires an 'open-minded' attitude and a willingness to discuss evidence-based practice with people who are enthusiastic about it. Greenhalgh (2014) identifies several **factors that influence an individual's readiness or motivation** to adopt an evidence-based approach. We summarize these as follows:

- Personality traits such as motivation and willingness to try out and use new things – if someone is 'set in their ways', they may be less likely to embrace EBP.
- An intervention that meets an identified need is more likely to be accepted.
- The decision to implement something new is rarely made in isolation. It is likely that discussion with others might influence a long-held belief about the need for change.

- The adoption of new practices is complex and will bring challenges at different stages. At first, professionals need general information about the nature of the evidence for change and associated costs. Later, they will need practical information about how to implement change.

Skills and competence

Leach and Gillham (2008) have identified the **skills needed** by individuals to implement an evidence-based approach in their EBASE tool. These include the ability to:

- Identify knowledge gaps in nursing practice
- Identify answerable clinical questions
- Locate professional literature
- Undertake a database search
- Retrieve evidence.

Leung et al. (2016) also developed a detalied set of **competencies** required by professionals when adopting an evidence-based approach based on the 5 steps of EBP!

- Ask
- Acquire
- Appraise
- Apply
- Assess (evaluate).

Melnyk et al. (2014, 2016a) have developed the following evidence-based practice competencies for implementing an evidence-based approach. We have adapted them to apply to all health and social care professionals.

Evidence-based practice competencies

Professionals should be able to:

1 Question practice with the aim of improving quality.
2 Describe clinical problems using evidence such as patient/client assessment, evaluation of outcomes and quality improvement information.
3 Formulate focused clinical questions using 'PICOT'.
4 Search for research evidence to answer focused clinical questions.
5 Critically appraise evidence from clinical practice guidelines, policies and procedures, and evidence summaries.

6   Critically appraise published research studies for quality and applicability to practice.

7   Evaluate and consider all the evidence for quality and applicability to practice.

8   Systematically collect practice data (such as individual patient and quality improvement data) for decision-making in relation to the care of individuals and groups.

9   Pull together all the evidence gathered, so as to plan evidence-based practice changes.

10 Implement change based on the evidence, clinical expertise, and patient preferences in order to improve care and outcomes.

11 Evaluate the outcomes of decisions and practice changes on individuals and groups to ascertain best practices.

12 Share best evidence-based practices.

13 Take part in strategies that help to maintain an evidence-based practice culture.

Assessing your motivation, attitude, skills, and competence

You might be interested in using **assessment tools** in relation to your own **attitude, skills, and competence in relation to evidence-based practice**. Tests are available to measure different aspects of evidence-based practice, many of which have been developed since the 'Sicily statement on classification and development of evidence-based practice learning assessment tools' (Tilson et al. 2011). Their consensus paper offers detailed guidance for the clear development of EBP assessment tools and principles and priorities. Many researchers have gone on to use a range of tools before and/or after educational interventions.

In relation to using a tool to assess **readiness or attitudes**, Leach et al. (2016) researched attitudes using the Evidence-Based Practice Attitude and Utilization Survey (EBASE) (developed by Leach and Gillham 2008), which asks practitioners to indicate on a 5-point Likert scale to what extent they agree with a number of statements about attitudes to evidence-based practice:

1   *EBP is necessary in the practice of nursing*
2   *Professional literature and research findings are useful in my day-to-day practice*
3   *I am interested in learning or improving the skills necessary to incorporate EBP into my practice*
4   *EBP improves the quality of my patient's care*
5   *EBP assists me in making decisions about patient care*

6 *EBP takes into account my clinical experience when making clinical decisions*

7 *EBP takes into account a patient's preference for treatment*

8 *The adoption of EBP places an unreasonable demand on my practice*

9 *There is a lack of evidence from clinical trials to support most of the treatments I use in my practice.*

(Leach et al. 2016: 199)

Leach and colleagues' (2016) participants had generally positive attitudes towards evidence-based practice before the intervention, which was an undergraduate research education programme, with most 'strongly agreeing' that EBP is necessary for practice and that it improves care. However, responses to only four of the nine statements (above) improved slightly following the intervention. The authors explain that this may be due to the learners already having a positive attitude, the quality of the educational programme or individual factors. This indicates the complexicity of assessing EBP.

Ilic et al. (2014) provide a useful overview of several tools that can be used for assessing your own **competence in evidence-based practice**. One of which was the 15-item Assessing Competence in Evidence Based Medicine (AE) tool, which assesses the main stages of the EBP process except for implementation. They found it to be reliable and valid in assessing medical trainees' competence. It also provided an assessment of deep learning, measuring the ability to ask, acquire, appraise, and apply evidence using a realistic patient scenario.

Greenhalgh (2014) has also developed a **self-assessment** tool to assess the use of evidence in practice and identify **gaps in knowledge**. This highlights the importance of thinking broadly and critically about our patient/client encounters. The following is a simplified version of Greenhalgh's (2014: Appendix 1) checklist, 'Is my practice evidence-based?'

Do you:

1 Identify and prioritize all the patient/client problem(s), including their own perspective?

2 Fully consider alternative diagnoses (not just medical ones)?

3 Deal with any additional problems and risk factors?

4 Seek best available evidence relating to the problems?

5 Fully appraise the evidence (amount and quality)?

6 Apply valid and relevant evidence to the problems logically and intuitively?

7 Present the options to the patient in a balanced, understandable way incorporating their preferences?

8 Arrange ongoing referral, evaluation, re-assessment or future care as need be?

Take a more detailed look at some of the EBP assessment tools and try to identify an area of your practice that you could develop.

There are many tools that help you assess your competence and willingness to promote EBP. In order to improve your skills you can also do the following:

- Discuss with your peers how confident they are in their practice knowledge (it is likely that some will feel the same as you).
- Participate in local or online journal clubs if offered by your organization – or initiate one yourself.
- Discuss at your performance management meeting any professional development needs you have in relation to searching for or appraising information and ensure your manager knows where you lack knowledge for your practice.
- Find out if your organization or library offers any face-to-face or online training or tutorials on evidence-based practice.
- Access high-quality video resources from YouTube or an online free course such as a Massive Open Online Course (MOOC), but make sure they are from reputable authors or organizations.
- Don't wait until you need the skills of evidence-based practice (for a course or a project) before you learn them. There will be greater pressure on you then.
- Practise searching for evidence using professional databases when you write an academic assignment rather than relying on the reference list or broad Internet searches.
- Read research and EBP research books and/or do online tutorials (see above) so that you become more familiar with the language and terminology used.

Use a **glossary** (there is one at the back of this book, or see the following online glossaries):

http://community-archive.cochrane.org/glossary,
https://www.nice.org.uk/glossary?letter=r
http://www.cebm.net/glossary/
http://jamaevidence.mhmedical.com/glossary.aspx
http://clinicalevidence.bmj.com/x/set/static/ebm/toolbox/678178.html

- See if there is a team member or student on placement who has more skill in searching and appraising than you and and ask them to help help you develop these skills.

- See if there are any EBP mentors in your organization; Melnyk et al. (2016) discuss the value of EBP mentors.
- Consider following professional journals on social media – many discuss EBP topics. WeCommunities organizes Twitter chats [see http://www.wecommunities.org/] and #WeCats organizes critical appraisal of papers via Twitter [see http://www.casp-uk.net/wecats].
- **Have a go!** Use widely available sites such as: http://www.cochranelibrary.com/ http://www.campbellcollaboration.org/ http://www.evidence.nhs.uk/ and just play around to see what is available.
- See the Appendix for **useful websites** for EBP resources and you may want to look within your own profession for **specific evidence-based practice journals.**

Moving on from an individual perspective, we need to look at the influence of the wider organization because although as individuals we can make a difference, together with colleagues we can have a greater impact.

Organizational culture

Although promoting an evidence-based approach requires commitment and implementation at an individual level, this alone is not enough. The research we have mentioned above has identified the challenges of getting evidence into practice, and from this it is clear that an organizational commitment is also required. Anyone who intends to influence organizational culture in relation to EBP needs to understand the factors that influence not only individual change but organizational change too (for a good overview of the factors, see Melnyk 2016b).

For an EBP culture to exist, a desire is needed across the organization for it to succeed – this requires motivation, openness to learning, infrastructure, leadership, and a willingness to provide resources and structures that support the uptake of evidence-based practice. Melnyk et al. (2016b: 11) assert:

> It is not enough to disseminate evidence-based guidelines and expect clinicians to readily implement them. For many clinicians, EBP requires behavior change from practice steeped in tradition and organizational cultures of 'this is the way we do it here' to practice that is supported by science.

An organizational culture of EBP is central to supporting sustainable high quality evidence-based care (Melnyk et al. 2016).

Melnyk (2016b: 99) notes that culture is frequently defined as 'the beliefs, behaviors, and values of people within an organization'.

It is widely recognized that organizational culture will influence the way in which evidence-based practice develops. Organizational culture is the factor that rises to the top in building and sustaining EBP context (Rycroft-Malone et al. 2013). Melnyk (2016b) recognizes that changing a culture often takes many years and requires a clear team vision, persistence, and patience. Therefore, knowing the stages of organizational change is essential when shifting culture in order to avoid the early discontinuation of one's efforts.

As a response to the need to focus on getting evidence into practice, the Promoting Action on Research Implementation in Health Services (PARIHS) framework was published in 1998. PARIHS was one of the first frameworks to recognize the multidimensional and complex nature of implementation of evidence-based practice, as well as highlight the central importance of contextual influences (Harvey and Kitson 2016).

As a result, a lot of work has explored what organizations can do to promote a culture of evidence-based practice. There is no single way to promote organizational willingness to promote evidence-based practice and many approaches have been piloted. These involve the use of mentors who facilitate the use of evidence within an organization (Kim et al. 2013; Melynk et al. 2017) and the promotion of accessible web-based materials (Glegg et al. 2016).

 Can you find any primary research on the specific implementation of evidence in your own profession or specialty?

Some evaluations of strategies used to implement evidence-based practice

Murthy et al. (2012) explored how the findings of systematic reviews could be implemented in practice. In a Cochrane review entitled 'Interventions to improve the use of systematic reviews in decision-making by health system managers, policy makers and clinicians', Murthy et al. concluded that 'mass mailing' a printed bulletin that summarizes the best available evidence can improve uptake of evidence-based practice in certain conditions: when there is a single clear message, if the change is relatively simple to accomplish, and there is a growing awareness by users of the evidence that a change in practice is required.

In another systematic review, Baker et al. (2015) updated an existing review to explore interventions that change professional practice. They found that tailored interventions – interventions that are planned in response to previous evaluations of barriers to change – can sometimes change professional practice in small to moderate ways. They noted that there is not enough evidence on the effectiveness and cost-effectiveness of such approaches and recommended further research.

In another Cochrane review, Flodgren et al. (2015) investigated the acceptability of tools to facilitate the dissemination of guidelines. They found that, in some specific areas, implementation tools developed by recognized guideline producers probably lead to an improvement in healthcare professionals' adherence to guidelines.

Regarding the current interest in childhood obesity, a Cochrane review by Wolfenden et al. (2016) highlight that 'little guidance is available for policy makers and practitioners interested in supporting the implementation of healthy eating, physical activity or obesity prevention policies, practices and programmes in centre-based childcare services'. They conclude that current research provides weak and inconsistent evidence of the effectiveness of the strategies to improve the implementation of policies and practices and so further research is needed.

There is no easy fix for getting evidence into practice. Reflect on an occasion when you tried to implement a change in practice and which factors had an effect on this.

These examples prove that getting evidence into practice is not an easy task. Further research is needed to explore strategies that will facilitate putting evidence into practice. This is supported by Melnyk, who notes:

> . . . *what is urgently needed are more high-quality intervention studies focused on overcoming those barriers and implementing strategies to enhance an EBP culture in real-world clinical settings.*
>
> (Melnyk 2016b)

Note that lack of evidence *does not mean that these organizational approaches don't work; it is just that we don't yet have the evidence and that further research is needed.*

Does your organization have an EBP culture?

There is an Organizational Culture and Readiness Scale for System-Wide Integration of Evidence-Based Practice (OCRSIEP) (Fineout-Overholt and Melnyk 2006). This instrument contains 26 Likert scale items relating to existing support for evidence-based practice within the current culture, offering insight into the strengths and opportunities for fostering evidence-based care within a healthcare system.

Leaders, experts, role models, and specialists

Leaders, experts, role models, and specialists may also be influential in leading and developing an evidence-based approach within an organization. There is some evidence to suggest that a senior member of staff's support for evidence-based practice will facilitate its development. Melnyk et al. (2016b: 12) note that transformation to an EBP culture requires:

> ... an exciting team vision and clear expectations from healthcare leaders that EBP is the foundation of all care delivered within the healthcare system. This expectation should be integrated into the vision, mission, and strategic plan of the institution and incorporated into the onboarding of all new clinicians.

Having someone in a senior position within the organization to promote evidence-based practice can influence its use (Sredl 2011; Greenhalgh 2014). Experts and specialists may be accessed through personal contacts, networking, and specialist interest groups in addition to their professional role. Such experts may have access to colleagues who may be able to reach agreed decisions on what is best practice. There are many published **consensus statements**. These papers can capture knowledge and skills that come from a vast range of practical experience in the field. For example, Young et al. (2016) produced 'Recommendations for the transition of patients with ADHD from child to adult healthcare services: a consensus statement from the UK adult ADHD network'.

Examples of studies that have identified the positive role of 'champions, mentors, experts, and specialists'

Titler et al. (2016) describe a variety of interventions including the use of 'change champions' to promote use of evidence-based fall prevention interventions in hospitalized adults in the USA.

The Advancing Research and Clinical practice through close Collaboration (ARCC) model is a system-wide model to advance and sustain evidence-based practice in healthcare system. Melnyk et al. (2017: 8) conclude that 'a key strategy in the ARCC model is the development of a critical mass of EBP mentors who assist point of care clinicians in the consistent implementation of evidence-based care', and that these mentors enhance professionals' beliefs and implementation of EBP and strengthen the EBP culture of an organization.

Harvey and Kitson (2015b, 2016) emphasize the role of facilitation in the implementation of evidence-based practice. They see facilitation as a mechanism for enabling change and development. They discuss the I-PARIHS framework and note that people rarely use a systematic review or clinical guideline in its original form but instead use evidence in a variety of ways, adapting it to suit the context. They see their I-PARIHS framework as a spiral indicating the dynamic nature of implementation. It starts by focusing on the innovation and the recipients, then moves to a local, organizational context, and then to a wider system and policy level.

Gerrish et al. (2011) presents a case study of 23 advanced practice nurses (APNs) from hospital and primary care settings across seven Strategic Health Authorities in England. She found that APNs promoted evidence-based practice among clinical nurses. They generated different types of evidence, accumulated evidence for clinical nurses, synthesized different forms of evidence, translated evidence by evaluating, interpreting and distilling it, and disseminated evidence in a variety of ways.

It is encouraging that expert and specialist roles may provide a platform for practitioners to have a real influence on decision-making. Such roles include consultant roles, specialist practitioners, specialists or leads in education and professional development. However, it is important to note that some experienced professionals may have never had any training or education in the knowledge and skills needed for evidence-based practice. It might sometimes be appropriate for a student to become a role model for the experienced professional, which relies on the professional being open to learning about new evidence and not feeling threatened by being challenged about the way he or she does things by a student, which we discuss further later in this chapter.

There is an important (if obvious) point to be made here:

Learning from experts (role modelling) only works well if the role model draws on current evidence-based information and research to inform their practice.

Clearly, if we role-model unsafe or out-of-date practices, ritualistic practice can thrive (as discussed in Chapter 2). If practitioners are not up to date, this is likely to have a big influence on colleague and student learning. There is the potential for practice to be based on ritual rather than evidence if both students and practitioners fail to be open to challenge in their practice.

What is the role of education in promoting an evidence-based approach?

What the role of education is in developing a culture in which evidence-based practice can thrive is yet to be established. Although there is evidence that those who have recently qualified, have advanced degrees or are in leadership roles are more likely to have a positive attitude towards evidence-based practice and embedding it into the organizational culture (Warren et al. 2016), information on how to implement such an approach is inconclusive, partly due to a lack of evidence. For example, Hecht et al. (2016) carried out a systematic review of the effects of evidence-based medicine (EBM) training for healthcare professionals. They concluded that there was insufficient evidence about the effect of training on the practice of professionals. They noted that future trials should focus not only on participants' knowledge, attitudes, and skills but address whether such courses lead to changes in care processes or patient-relevant outcomes.

Yost et al. (2014) also reported that research has focused on the development of search and appraisal skills rather than the actual implementation of evidence. They developed an Evidence Informed Decision Making (EIDM) tool that assesses the relevance of evidence in relation to decision-making in specific scenarios. They found that a one-week educational workshop promoted the lasting retention of knowledge and skills among a broad range of health professionals, but did not result in significant behaviour change.

Crabtree et al. (2012) used the Adapted Fresno Test (AFT) to explore whether skills and knowledge were improved following an EBP course. They found that while skills improved, these were not retained for use in practice. The shortened Adapted Fresno Test (SAFT) has proved useful in circumstances where evidence-based practice is an emerging approach and time is at a premium (Buchanan et al. 2015).

These studies indicate that the relationship between knowledge and skills and the implementation of an evidence-based approach in practice is not linear. The predominant view from many studies is that following educational intervention, knowledge and skills do not always translate into use of evidence in practice and indeed positive patient/client outcomes. More strategies and research are therefore needed.

If you are an educationalist or practice mentor/supervisor, a variety of techniques are useful for keeping evidence-based practice at the forefront of the minds of students throughout the curriculum. Based on a systematic review of educational interventions to teach evidence-based practice, Kyriakoulis et al. (2016) found that a multi-methods approach to activities and strategies to promote EBP was needed if students were to remain interested in it. They also found that technology to promote evidence based practice through mobile devices, simulation, and the web is on the increase, although not yet evaluated.

You can help develop the skills and knowledge of, as well as a positive attitude towards evidence-based practice in others in the following ways:

- Ensure that the skills, knowledge, and attitude required for evidence-based practice are clear in the learning outcomes of courses or practice activities.
- Introduce evidence-based practice early on in the curriculum.
- Offer regular, timetabled library skills sessions.
- Ensure that clinical/professional skills sessions have a clear evidence-based and relevant research is available for students.
- State clearly when there is a lack of evidence or it is inconclusive.
- Invite practitioners to contribute (as facilitators or patients) in the simulated learning environment.
- Ensure that evidence-based practice is related explicitly to decision-making to ensure that students are more likely to engage with it.
- Make the use of evidence and critical appraisal evident in the grading criteria and in both academic and practice-based assignments (competencies).
- Encourage students to use subject librarians and study skills support available at the university.
- Ensure that role modelling and evidence-based practice are discussed as part of practice educator update days.
- Ensure learners have an opportunity to discuss what to do if they see practices that are not evidence-based.
- Encourage lecturers to make explicit how the research that underpins teaching is appraised (so they role-model critical appraisal in their teaching).

Finding solutions to the problems of implementing evidence-based practice

We have looked at the role of both the individual and the organization in the implementation of evidence-based practice. Given that, even at organizational level, attitudes and approaches to evidence-based practice are influenced by individuals, it is possible to conclude that it is the individual who is critical in promoting an evidence-based approach. In relation to the **barriers to implementing evidence-based practice** introduced earlier, we have developed the following six strategies that can be adopted by individuals at every level within an organization to promote an evidence-based approach.

Strategy 1: Develop your understanding of research papers

This book has provided you with a 'Beginner's guide to evidence-based practice'. We have explored how to search for high-quality evidence; if you are a student, your course will undoubtedly cover this in detail – so do make the most of the practice and library sessions you are allocated. Once you have grasped the main concepts, you may want to access a wider range of sources and higher-level reading to improve your understanding of research and evidence-based practice.

 If you are a qualified practitioner, seek opportunities to learn how to search for evidence and ask your students to help you if you remain unsure. It is good practice for them and you!

We have addressed how to critically appraise the research and have suggested the use of specific and general appraisal tools and checklists. We recommend that initially you use our **Six Questions to Trigger Critical Thinking** (Aveyard et al. 2015) when you hear, see or read something that relates to your practice. We do not recommend that you attempt to understand every word of a research paper. Many people struggle with understanding the results when they are presented as statistics; indeed, many researchers use statisticians to help them design and interpret their studies (we provide several glossaries and helpful websites that can help you understand statistical findings). However, you should be able to understand the main points in a paper. You should also read the discussion part of the research or, if it is a systematic review, see if they have a plain language summary of the paper to more easily explain their findings. Try and learn about some of the common phrases you read as you develop as an evidence-based practitioner.

Strategy 2: Develop the practical skill of searching

Literature searching in a systematic and thorough way is a skill that takes practice. We would strongly recommend that you practise the skills of formulating a focused question, searching using Boolean operators and truncation in order to become proficient. We have emphasized the importance of systematic reviews and good literature reviews that summarize the available evidence on a topic. You will find it easier if it is something you find interesting and it is highly relevant to your practice.

If a literature search fails to identify any reviews, consider whether you could undertake a review yourself with the help of your colleagues, or if you are about to commence an academic course of study, consider whether you could undertake a review as a component of your course.

Part of being accountable for safe and effective practice is to recognize and address any limitations in your knowledge and skills and seek further education.

Strategy 3: Increase your engagement with research

Promoting evidence-based practice is about promoting the appropriate use of research as an individual and within your organization. We have addressed this throughout this book. You may have never studied research methods or been taught how to adopt a critical approach to literature – this will depend on where or when you began your training. However, as evidence-based practice is a requirement of all health and social care professions, we all need to share our expertise and experience in professional practice.

If you supervise students, find out what evidence they are using on their course. They have access to up-to-date lectures, seminars, and library resources (many of which may be online) and you may be able to learn from them.

Make the most of educational and development opportunities offered within your working day. Attend journal clubs, in-house training, and seminars on offer, even if you do not feel that you can contribute much. Many learning resources are available online, meaning that you can access them at any time (e.g. webinars, MOOCs, blogs, catching up on professional social media accounts and professionally produced video). You will soon realize that you have a useful contribution to make.

Scurlock-Evans et al. (2014) explored interventions for increasing the practical/applied value of research among physiotherapists. They found the following helpful:

- Increasing open-access resources and peer-reviewed 'coffee table' publications in an effort to reduce time and resource demands.

- Information-seeking from 'human' as opposed to 'computer' sources was preferred.
- In-house CPD activities appear to be a key method of ensuring knowledge and skills remain current.
- Greater organizational commitment to key changes in policy, guidelines or research.

They note that a variety of approaches need to be adopted, as practitioners work in different settings, have different educational needs, and encounter different barriers.

Examples

McKeever et al. (2016) had more success with a journal club for paediatric nurses after introducing an element of competition. They also offered support for staff in understanding the suitability and results of the studies.

Ferguson et al. (2017) found that a social media-facilitated journal club was a good way of developing critical appraisal skills and it increased students' attention, engagement with presented activities, and overall satisfaction.

You could also set up email alerts on professional journal websites, whereby you will receive regular 'contents' updates of articles just published. It is best to do this with journals that are open access or that you or your organization subscribe to – this way you will be able to access the full-text version of the paper.

Strategy 4: Use evidence-based guidelines, policy, summaries or syntheses of evidence

As busy practitioners, it is important to be focused in how we use our time. As part of our working day, we are unlikely to be able to stop what we are doing and carry out a literature search! Thus, we need to be aware of how we can access information that has already been summarized or synthesized for us. Some of this information may be local and produced by your own organization. You will of course need to check the sources are up to date.

There is a move worldwide to provide 'synthesized evidence' that is readily available to practitioners.

These can be in a variety of forms, including **evidence-based** . . .

- guidelines
- policy
- care pathways
- clinical knowledge summaries
- websites offering access to synthesized evidence (you can search for 'evidence summaries' or see our useful websites section)
- plain language summaries of systematic reviews – see Cochrane Library [http://www.cochranelibrary.com/].

There is recognition that providing accessible, synthesized summaries of evidence may be a better way of getting evidence into practice for busy professionals.

Using guidelines, policy, and care pathways

Remind yourself, by reading Chapter 4, about using evidence-based guidelines and policy as a more accessible form of evidence for your practice. According to Van Beek et al. (2016), who carried out a European-wide systematic review to assess the integration of palliative care in the content of guidelines/pathways of adult cancer patients in Europe, a **care pathway** is 'a complex intervention for the mutual decision making and organisation of care processes for a well-defined group of patients during a well-defined period' (p. 26).

Greenhalgh (2014) suggests a range of reasons for using guidelines, such as cost-effectiveness, objective decision-making, and education purposes. She notes that many clinicians are reluctant to use guidelines for various reasons, including practicality and acceptability. She defines **guidelines** as 'systematically developed statements to assist practitioner decisions about appropriate health care for specific clinical circumstances' (p. 135).

In the UK, the National Institute for Health and Care Excellence (NICE) produces a wide range of guidelines [https://www.nice.org.uk/guidance], and takes into account the costs and benefits of interventions. Drummond (2016) notes that there is bound to be tension in advising on quality of care while recognizing the broader public health objectives of equity, fairness, and efficiency.

Policies or **protocols** may also be used within professional organizations and as employees we will be accountable to the organization for adherence to these documents. There may be delays between the recognition of new evidence and a change to policy/protocols within an organization and how that would impact on the accountability of a professional.

Resources for evidence synthesis, guidelines, and pathways

NICE CKS provides an accessible summary of the current evidence base and practical guidance on best practice in respect of over 330 common and/or significant primary care presentations [https://cks.nice.org.uk/#?char=A]. NICE has also produced PowerPoint slides that can be used as an educational tool [https://cks.nice.org.uk/slides].

The Centre for Research and Dissemination (CRD) has an evidence synthesis centre that summarizes evidence in formats that are accessible to health and social care decision-makers [https://www.york.ac.uk/crd/research/service-delivery/york-evidence-synthesis-centre/].

The National Elf Service has summaries of evidence and blogs for social work, mental health, learning disabilities, social care, and musculoskeletal issues [https://www.nationalelfservice.net/].

The National Institute of Health Research (NIHR) provides select evidence synthesis [https://www.journalslibrary.nihr.ac.uk/search/#/?search=evidence%20synthesis&sitekit=true&indexname=fullindex&task=search&selected_facets=].

NICE Pathways is a key resource for NICE guidance [https://www.nice.org.uk/About/What-we-do/Our-Programmes/About-NICE-Pathways].

The Care Quality Commission's (CQC) 'Looking at the quality of care pathways' addresses how well the 'system' delivers joined-up care [http://www.cqc.org.uk/what-we-do/coordinated-care/looking-quality-care-pathways].

Public Health England has produced population screening pathways [https://www.gov.uk/government/collections/nhs-population-screening-care-pathways].

Remember to critically appraise guidelines as explored in Chapter 6, as they may not be evidence-based or up to date.

We discuss using specific databases in detail in Chapter 5. In the Appendix, we offer some broader resources that offer collections and synthesis of evidence.

Try accessing some of the websites offered in the Appendix and see which ones you find useful for your particular profession and specialty.

Strategy 5: Make the most of your time

Being under-staffed, too busy, and unable to get all our work done are constant issues in most health and social care workers' lives. Time management is widely discussed in the literature and strategies are offered to help us manage our time better. It is therefore worth thinking about ways and means of incorporating evidence in our practice in a more time-effective way. Guides to help us prioritize sometimes offer the idea that we should consider what is **urgent** and **important** when making priority decisions. There are also resources that can help save time such as systematic reviews, guidelines, care pathways, and synthesized knowledge summaries. Consider the time that will be saved if there is a **clear and consistent approach** to care that will result in the best outcomes for your patients/clients.

Time is our most precious resource and busy practitioners 'keep their heads down' and do what they need to do to get the job done. Evidence-based practice seems to be an optional extra. This then becomes a wider organizational issue where strong leadership has the potential to encourage change. Managers should ensure that **staffing levels allow time for developing and implementing an evidence-based approach** to practice. This then shows that professional development is valued within the organization.

Try considering the following:

- Do what you can to make evidence-based practice a part of your daily routine rather than an add-on.
- Use research-based activities as evidence if you have to 'revalidate' for your profession or if you have to produce evidence for your appraisal or performance review.
- For when things are less busy, have articles, guidelines, and other evidence ready to read.
- See if you can network with others in similar specialities so that you can combine your efforts.
- Develop a questioning culture so you can share information with colleagues.
- Agree that you will ask each other why you approach a task or intervention in a particular way and try and find out if there is any evidence for that approach.
- Ask any students you have on placement to talk about what they are learning in university (ask them to bring in relevant articles/lecture notes or even make a presentation to the team).
- See if your student has time/need to investigate a specific issue and whether they would be interested in doing a literature review on a topic relevant to your practice.

- Ask experts/specialists for any summaries/guidelines they know of relating to your speciality (remember to critically appraise them).
- Start by accessing sites that contain systematic reviews or knowledge summaries or evidence-based practice journals rather than individual articles or books.
- Take turns to find out the best available evidence on a topic and present it at team meetings.
- Ensure any staff member who attends a study day/conference or course feeds back to the wider team any implications for practice.
- Try and build in the evidence base for your other priorities (targets, projects or strategies) and see how it relates to improving patient/client outcomes.
- Consider if attending a clinical/professional conference or doing a course would be a faster/more effective way of ensuring your practice is up to date.

Strategy 6: Develop authority and confidence to influence and obtain resources and support

Some of these areas may be outside your control, but think about what you can do. Consider if you have communicated any resource/support needs in a constructive and assertive way. Talk to colleagues and see if they feel the same and find someone with influence to act on your behalf. Your own confidence will develop as you become more knowledgeable about research and evidence-based practice.

We have discussed how leadership can have an impact on the adoption of evidence-based practice. If the leader in your workplace is unsupportive, you may have to develop wider support from networking and from colleagues further afield such as experts. Ask yourself why some colleagues may be unsupportive of evidence-based practice – is it because they are under pressure themselves, are threatened by change or may not see what you want to do as a priority? Communication is the key! Ask them what their reasons are and try to explore a solution together – compromise is often the answer.

Challenging our own practice and that of others

As we discussed earlier, it is hard to leave behind practices that we are familiar and comfortable with. One of the reasons that students and qualified practitioners are reluctant to bring in new ideas is a **fear of challenging the status quo**, although in the UK professional body standards do outline professionals' responsibility in responding to unsafe practice (which may be the case if the care is not evidence-based). The Health and Care Professions Council's (HCPC 2016: 8) 'Standards of Conduct, Performance and Ethics' state that:

> You must not do anything, or allow someone else to do anything, which could put the health or safety of a service user, carer or colleague at unacceptable risk.

The Nursing and Midwifery Council (NMC 2015b:1 2) in its professional standards of practice and behaviour for nurses and midwives states that as a nurse you have a duty to

> ... raise and, if necessary, escalate any concerns you may have about patient or public safety, or the level of care people are receiving in your workplace or any other healthcare setting and use the channels available to you in line with our guidance and your local working practices.

Our students often tell us that they try and share with their practice assessors/mentors things they have learnt but are met with a defensive or reluctant response rather than an open and interested attitude.

Think about how you and your team react to having your practice challenged. Is it seen as a way of professionally developing or as a personal criticism? Could you do more to invite challenge to your practice – give permission for others to question you?

Most people would welcome feedback to improve their practice, although it is worth remembering that in a busy working environment our natural reaction is likely to be defensive, especially if practice is challenged in an insensitive way; being tactful might prevent a 'defensive response'. However, you are accountable for your own practice and you may have to be assertive. For more about this, do look at the Royal College of Nursing's (RCN 2014) 'Good practice for handling feedback' [see https://www.rcn.org.uk/professional-development/publications/pub-004725].

Example

It is easier to propose a change in practice if you are sure about the evidence underpinning any such change and can produce the source of that evidence.

Think of an occasion when someone challenged you about something that was entirely justifiable. If they approached you in a tactful way, you would probably have been more likely to accept what they were saying than if they confronted you directly.

Ideas for adopting a more open approach to challenging practice

- Discuss in advance with colleagues/practice educators/students what you should do if you see practice that conflicts with evidence you are aware of.
- Before you challenge the practice of others, consider the validity of the evidence you have – *might there be things you are unaware of, for example, context, more than one approach or different values?*
- Try and start a conversation with someone and ask tactfully about the evidence underpinning some decision.
  - ○ Ask for their perspective on the issue/your observations.
  - ○ Offer to share that you have just found a new way of doing something.
  - ○ Ask if you can help to find the evidence for a particular therapy or intervention.
  - ○ Consider asking questions rather than making accusations about practice.
  - ○ Give them time to consider your view or question.
  - ○ Suggest the issue as a topic for a journal club or team project.
- Consider if the practice is unsafe or inappropriate; your role might be as an advocate for your patients or clients – this may help you to be assertive.
- Consider the setting; avoid challenging another practitioner in public unless the practice is unsafe. Ask to speak to them privately.

 Consider what you would do if you spotted unsafe or out-of-date practice by a colleague, practice educator or student.

 For very user-friendly guides on challenging poor practice, see the booklets and scenarios published by **Dignity in Care** (2014) [http://www.dignityincare.org.uk/Resources/resource/?cid=8227].

NHS employers have a series of resources and materials that organizations can display, and provide links to other **professional bodies'** guides and advice [see http://www.nhsemployers.org/your-workforce/retain-and-improve/raising-concerns-at-work-and-whistleblowing].

See information about raising and escalating concerns from the **HCPC** (2017) [http://www.hpc-uk.org/registrants/raisingconcerns/] and the **NMC** (2015c) [https://www.nmc.org.uk/standards/guidance/raising-concerns-guidance-for-nurses-and-midwives/].

Adopting some of these approaches may help you to move away from ritualistic or routine approaches to professional practice towards a more evidence-based approach.

The future of evidence-based practice

A variety of views are being debated in the literature regarding the value of evidence-based practice and its role as part of a wider spectrum of the art, values, and science of professional health and social care. These sometimes diverse but often overlapping views are a valuable part of a healthy debate ensuring the focus for practitioners is on delivery of a safe, effective, and compassionate health and social care. There is undoubtedly more work to do in the education of practitioners to develop the knowledge, skills, and positive attitudes towards searching and appraising evidence so it can be used alongside clinical/professional judgement and patient/client preferences in their decision-making.

There is an increasing emphasis on overcoming barriers and finding a range of ways to successfully implement evidence into practice and evaluate these approaches and the positive outcomes for patients/clients. Although there is widespread reporting of context-specific examples, there is clearly need for more high-quality and wider-reaching research.

In summary

Throughout this book we have shown that developing an EBP approach is both a personal and an organizational responsibility. As an individual, it is vital that you understand why evidence-based practice is an important aspect of delivering safe and effective practice. All practitioners need to be aware of the need for evidence-based practice and to have the skills to search for, evaluate, and understand the evidence they find. Adoption of an evidence-based approach is more likely if you are working within an organizational culture that is open and receptive to change and is prepared to embrace the concept of using evidence in practice. But remember that the culture of an organization is dependent on the individuals within it. There is much that you as an individual alongside your colleagues can do to support the development of this culture, as outlined in this chapter. There is increased recognition of the value of synthesized resources to help individual practitioners and organizations.

We hope that you have found this introduction to evidence-based practice useful and relevant to your professional lives.

Key points

1 Developing evidence-based practice requires practitioners to have the skills of finding and evaluating evidence.
2 This requires the motivation and dedication of the individual practitioner to achieve this.
3 Developing an EBP approach also requires an open and supportive organizational culture willing to adopt change.
4 Remember that the organization is made up of individuals, so do not underestimate your own contribution to the organizational culture – even as a student.
5 There is increasing recognition that synthesized evidence such as that in systematic reviews, evidence synthesis, policy and guidelines can help busy practitioners, but more research is clearly needed.

Quiz questions

1 Provide at least four reasons why it is challenging to get evidence into practice.
2 What five skills might you need to adopt an evidence-based approach?
3 Discuss at least four strategies you yourself could use to get more evidence into practice.

Glossary

Note that some words spelt with a 'z' can take an 's' in the UK, for example 'randomize' can also be spelt 'randomised'.

For **any terms not in this glossary**, please see our **Index** or the **Appendix**, which provides information on online glossaries.

Abstract: A summary of a research or discussion paper. The abstract will give you a general overview of the paper but you are advised to access the whole paper if it is of interest to you.

Action research: A study carried out in a practical setting, often involving those working there with the intent of introducing change. The results are implemented and evaluated within that setting.

Anonymity: Ensuring the identity of research participants is kept secret, so that they cannot be linked with the data (participants are often given numbers or pseudonyms).

Applicability: Whether the findings of a study can be used in relation to patients/clients in a particular area.

Bias: Flaws in the design or conduct of a study that can lead to the wrong result.

Blinding: An approach used when either the participants or researchers (or both in the case of double blinding) are unaware of the full details of the study. Blinding is used to reduce bias when awareness of some aspect of the study would be likely to affect behaviour.

Campbell Collaboration: A worldwide collaboration that commissions and maintains systematic reviews in social care.

Case control study: A study in which people with a specific condition (cases) are compared to people without this condition (controls) to compare the frequency of occurrence of the exposure that might have caused the disease.

Clinical practice guideline: A summary of current evidence to assist professionals make decisions about care.

Clinical trial: A study undertaken in a clinical area to compare the effects of an intervention. The term clinical trial is often used to refer to a randomized controlled trial.

Cochrane Collaboration: A worldwide collaboration that commissions and maintains systematic reviews in health care.

Coding: The process of giving a code to a piece of qualitative data in order to help with analysis. Codes are then combined into categories for further analysis.

Cohort study: A study in which two or more groups or cohorts are followed up to examine whether exposures measured at the beginning lead to outcomes, such as disease.

Concept analysis: A structured process by which complex or vague terms are defined by exploring predetermined aspects of the concept such as use, attributes, definitions, etc.

Confidence intervals: These express the uncertainty of our estimate. They use the result found in a study to make a prediction about what the 'true' result in the whole population might be.

Confirmability: In qualitative research, the extent to which the results can be confirmed or repeated in another experiment.

Confounding factors or variables: Other factors that may influence the results of a study – these can generally be eliminated by randomization.

CONSORT (Consolidated Standards of Reporting Trials) statement: A statement that describes the information that should be included in the report of a trial [see http://www.consort-statement.org/].

Content analysis: An in-depth examination of non-numerical data (i.e. words/text) to identify common content.

Control group: A group in an experiment or trial that does not receive the intervention/therapy or its members may receive a placebo.

Convenience sample: A sample that is obtained due to convenience factors – for example, all those attending a seminar are invited to complete a questionnaire.

Credibility: Evidence from the study that the results or conclusions are believable. Used in the evaluation of qualitative studies (see also *trustworthiness*).

Critical appraisal: A process by which the quality of evidence is assessed, evaluated or questioned in relation to quality and relevance – often using a critical appraisal tool.

Critical appraisal tool: A list of questions or checklist used to help assess the quality of evidence. It is often specific to the type of paper/ research.

Data analysis: The examination or interpretation of the data (results/ findings) collected in a study. Data are often analysed using thematic or statistical analysis.

Database: A collection of data. In research, a database normally refers to a collection of journals that are searchable electronically.

Dependability: Often used in qualitative research to describe whether the researcher accounts for the methods and results reported in the study, and the extent to which the reader can depend or rely on the results as presented.

Dependent variable: A variable that is dependent on the independent variable. It is generally the outcome of the intervention or therapy.

Descriptive (or narrative) review: An approach to undertaking a literature review, but not one that is undertaken according to a predefined or systematic approach.

Descriptive statistics: Statistics such as means, medians, and standard deviations that describe aspects of the data, such as central tendency (mean or median) or its dispersion (standard deviation).

Discourse analysis: An approach to the analysis of language use in order to understand meaning in complex areas.

Discussion paper: A paper presenting an argument or discussion that does not contain empirical research findings.

Dissemination: Ensuring that research is shared with a wider audience.

Double blind study: A study in which neither the researchers nor the participants are aware of which treatment or intervention the participants are receiving.

Effect size: The size of the effect – the difference between the intervention and the control group in an experiment. It is considered important alongside statistical significance (not just whether there is a difference but how big the difference is between the intervention and control).

Empirical research: Research carried out in the 'field' where data are collected first-hand. It is often based on observation or experiment and written up as a research study.

Ethnography: A qualitative research approach that involves the study of culture/way of life of participants.

Evidence-based practice: Practice based on the best available evidence, informed by patient preferences and clinical/professional judgement.

Exclusion criteria: Criteria about what or who will NOT be included in a research study or a literature search. (e.g. not children, not acute care episodes, literature not older than 5 years).

Experimental research: A study designed to test whether a treatment or intervention is effective.

Forest plot: A graph illustrating the spread of individual results combined in a meta-analysis. The plot displays the extent to which all the studies in a review have similar or dissimilar results.

Generalize: To apply the findings of one study to the wider population in other settings. Generalizability relates to quantitative research only, as qualitative studies do not seek to generalize (see *transferability*).

Gold standard: A procedure or method that is widely regarded as being the best available.

Grounded theory: A qualitative research approach that involves exploration of a topic about which little is known and results in the generation of theory.

Guideline: A systematically developed statement to assist practitioners in the delivery of evidence-based care. Guidelines should be evidence-based.

Hawthorne effect: A bias or change that may occur if participants are aware that they are being investigated.

Hierarchy of evidence: A grading system for ranking the best form of evidence to answer a specific question. Remember there is no one hierarchy of evidence – it all depends on the question!

Hypothesis: A statement or prediction drafted at the outset of a piece of research that the researchers try to prove or disprove (see also *null hypothesis*).

Incidence rate: The rate of occurrence that is measured within a set number of people and within a time period.

Inclusion criteria: Criteria chosen to determine what/who *will be* included in a research study or literature review (e.g. research from the past 5 years, published in the English language, women with depression). Usually reported alongside exclusion criteria.

Independent variable: A variable that is manipulated or studied in the research (such as an intervention or therapy).

Inferential statistics: Statistics that are used to apply findings from the sample population to the wider population, usually meaning statistical tests.

Informed consent: Written or verbal permission of an individual to participate in a study having been fully informed about the research.

Intervention: A treatment or therapy intended to improve or affect health or social care outcomes.

Intervention group: The group of participants within a experimental research study who receive the treatment or therapy.

Journal: An academic publication in which researchers publish their research. There are academic journals for many subjects and disciplines.

Keywords or key terms: Words or terms used when searching an electronic database for literature that represent the focus of the topic you wish to study. Academic papers entered into the database are indexed using keywords/key terms.

Limitations: A statement in a research paper (or literature review) where the authors identify any weaknesses in the research process that subsequently could affect the validity of the results.

Literature review: A collection of research papers and other evidence on a particular topic. A good literature (or systematic) review should let you know precisely how it was carried out, including how the quality of the papers was judged.

Matching: See *stratification.*

Mean: The average of a set of numbers that is calculated by adding up the individual scores and dividing by the number of people or items.

MeSH: Medical Subject Headings – a thesaurus of medical terms used to index medical information in some databases.

Meta-analysis: A process by which quantitative data (with similar properties) are combined to produce a weighted average of all the results.

Meta-ethnography: A process by which the results of qualitative data are combined.

Meta-study: A process by which the results of all types of data are combined.

Minimization: See *stratification.*

Mixed-methods: A research study that uses more than one approach to data collection (often a combination of quantitative and qualitative).

Narrative or descriptive review: An approach to undertaking a literature review, but not one that is undertaken according to a predefined or systematic approach.

Non-empirical evidence: Evidence that is not based on the findings of research.

Non-responder bias: Bias may be introduced if not all people respond to a questionnaire/survey. There may be a difference between those who did respond and those who didn't.

Null hypothesis: A statement (to be proved or disproved) that there is no relationship between the variables to be explored in the study.

Odds ratio: The odds of an event occurring in the experimental group, divided by the odds of an event occurring in the control group.

Outcome: The end result or consequence (of a study). The outcome is often the focal point of a study.

Peer review: The process in which experts in a subject area are invited to review the academic work of an author, often prior to publication in a journal.

Phenomenology: A qualitative research approach in which the participants' 'lived experience' is explored.

PICOT: Acronym used for forming a research question – Population, Intervention/Issue, Comparison/Context, Outcome and Time – sometimes shortened to **PICO.**

Placebo: In experimental research, a dummy or sham drug, treatment or intervention is given as a control to that which is being researched.

Primary research/research study: A study undertaken using a planned and methodological approach.

Probability: The likelihood or not of results occurring by chance. Is presented as p-values. The p-value is the probability of the difference between groups in an experiment being due to chance.

Professional judgement: Considered judgement made by a professional when making a decision. Professional judgement is a component of evidence-based practice.

Purposive sampling: Sampling strategy used by qualitative researchers when looking for a population that is 'fit for the purposes' of the study in question.

p-value: See *probability.*

Qualitative research: Research that involves an in-depth understanding of the experiences and meanings of human behaviour with the results presented in words.

Quantitative research: Research that involves collecting data that can be defined in categories and presented numerically.

Questionnaire: A list of questions to be asked of respondents, sometimes called a survey.

Quasi-experiment: A type of experimental study that doesn't meet all the requirements of a true experiment (usually randomization).

Randomization or random allocation: The process of allocating individuals at random (by chance) to groups, usually in a randomized controlled trial, to ensure that two or more groups in a trial are equal in terms of participants' characteristics.

Randomized controlled trial: A quantitative research approach that has randomly assigned groups in order to determine the effectiveness of interventions or therapies.

Random sampling: A sampling strategy in which everyone in a given population has an equal chance of being selected and that probability is independent of any other person selected.

Raw data: The primary data that have been gathered from participants such as physiological or psychological measurements, rankings or scores. In qualitative research, the written words (when transcribed).

Relevance: Research that can be applied to any patient or client group and context. A term often used in the evaluation of qualitative studies.

Reliability: The extent to which something measured is deemed consistent in a study and would be repeated if the study were to be conducted a second time.

Reproducibility: Being clearly described, the study as a whole, or in part, could be repeated in other settings by other people.

Research method: The tool or approach used to gather the data such as interview, experiment or survey.

Research methodology: The whole study process undertaken in order to address the research question – for example, randomized controlled trial, ethnographic study.

Research process: A systematic, thorough approach for undertaking a research study.

Research question: A question set at the outset of a study, to be addressed by the researchers during the study (see *PICOT*).

Research study/primary study: A study undertaken using a planned and methodological approach that includes a research question/aims, data collection, analysis, results and conclusions.

Response rate: The number of people who responded to a survey or questionnaire divided by the number of people who received the survey/questionnaire. This is usually presented as a percentage.

Review of research: A synthesis of research on a particular topic. If the review is not referred to as systematic, check to see if the method of undertaking the search is clearly defined – if it is not, it is likely to be less reliable.

Rigour: Assessment of the way in which a study has been undertaken. A rigorous study is one that has been carried out meticulously. A study that lacks rigour is one that is haphazard in design.

Risk ratio: The ratio of risk of an event occurring in the experimental group divided by the risk in the control group.

Ritualistic practice: Practice that is carried out as routine without question or an evidence base.

Sample: The group of people included in a study. This could be a random sample for a quantitative study, or a purposive or theoretical sample for a qualitative study. Some samples are convenience samples.

Search strategy: A planned strategy for searching the literature. A comprehensive search strategy is a component of undertaking a rigorous literature review.

Secondary source: A source that the reader has not accessed themselves – but has used someone else's representation or interpretation of it.

Shared decision-making: The active involvement of patients/clients in deciding treatment or therapy options using the best available evidence and, if relevant, decision-making tools or aids.

Snowball sampling: A sampling strategy in which who/what is involved in the study (sample) is determined according to the needs of the study as the investigation progresses.

Snowballing literature: An approach used to find more relevant research or information by using the reference lists of studies or papers already found (backward/reverse snowballing) or seeing where the given paper is cited (forward snowballing) to identify new sources.

Standard deviation: Shows how spread out the data are from the average (mean): the greater the spread of the data, the larger the standard deviation. If the deviation is small, then most results are close to the average. This is often represented in a distribution curve.

Statistical significance: A term used to indicate that a result is unlikely to be due to chance. Usually represented by a p-value.

Statistics: The collection, organization, and analysis of numerical data. Statistics are generally used in quantitative studies to represent the data collected. Two different types of statistics are commonly used in quantitative research: *descriptive* and *inferential statistics* (defined above).

Stratification: The sample is divided into groups that have the same value or characteristics, for example, stratifying by age means putting people of the same age or age group together. Sometimes done before randomization to avoid confounding variables.

Strengths: In the context of evidence-based practice, strengths refer to the positive points in a study that give the evidence more weight.

Systematic review: A very detailed review of the literature that is undertaken according to a defined and systematic approach. The way in which the review was carried out will be clearly detailed.

Theoretical sampling: An approach to sampling in grounded theory where the sampling strategy evolves as the study progresses, according to the needs of the study and the developing theory.

Transferability: Refers to the extent to which the results or findings of a study may be transferred to (or have meaning for) another context or population. Transferability is usually used in qualitative research where the aim is not to generalize, but to consider the extent to which significant concepts identified may be transferable to other contexts.

Triangulation: Use of several data collection or data analysis methods in a research study.

Trustworthiness: The honest and reliable reporting of a study, including credibility and dependability. This concept usually relates to qualitative studies.

Validity: The extent to which a study or an intervention measures what it intended to measure.

Variables: A set of attributes or qualities (see also *dependent variable* and *independent variable*).

Appendix: Useful websites and social media

All websites were accessed in April 2017 and were accurate at the time of going to press. If a link no longer works, a simple Internet search of the organization/title should enable you to access the appropriate website. Sites in boxes marked with two asterisks (**) are considered to be excellent general sites or gateways to other resources.

The sites are organized into the following sections:

- Online glossaries for research- and evidence-based practice terms
- General useful websites for evidence-based practice and finding evidence
- Appraisal tools/checklists
- Useful video/audio
- Professional bodies
- Social media

Online glossaries for research- and evidence-based practice terms

- Bandolier Glossary [http://www.bandolier.org.uk/glossary.html]
- BMJ Clinical Evidence Glossary [http://clinicalevidence.bmj.com/x/set/static/ebm/toolbox/678178.html]
- Centre for Evidence based Medicine Glossary [http://www.cebm.net/glossary/]
- Cochrane Glossary [http://community-archive.cochrane.org/glossary]
- CONSORT Glossary [http://www.consort-statement.org/resources/glossary]
- JAMA Evidence [http://jamaevidence.mhmedical.com/glossary.aspx]
- National Institute of Health Research Evaluation, Trials and Studies (NETS) [http://www.nets.nihr.ac.uk/glossary?result_1655_result_page=A]
- NICE Glossary [https://www.nice.org.uk/glossary?letter=r]

General useful websites for evidence-based practice and finding evidence

Bad Science: A website by columnist Ben Goldacre that offers a light-hearted view on health and social care stories from the media and wider afield [http://www.badscience.net/].

BestBets was developed to provide rapid evidence-based answers to real-life clinical questions, using a systematic approach to reviewing the literature [http://www.bestbets.org/].

Campbell Collaboration: The Campbell Collaboration promotes positive social and economic change through the production and use of systematic reviews and other evidence synthesis (plain language and policy briefs) for evidence-based policy and practice [http://www.campbellcollaboration.org/]. They also have a link to other **evidence portals relating to public health and social care [https://www.campbellcollaboration.org/better-evidence/evidence-portals.html].

Care Quality Commission (CQC): The independent regulator of health and social care in England [http://www.cqc.org.uk].

Centre for Evidence Based Interventions (CEBI): CEBI is a global leader in conducting rigorous evaluations of interventions aimed at tackling today's urgent social problems [https://www.cebi.ox.ac.uk/for-practitioners.html].

Centre for Evidence-Based Medicine (CEBM): CEBM aims to 'develop, teach and promote evidence-based healthcare through conferences, workshops and EBM tools so that all healthcare professionals can maintain the highest standards of medicine'. Online tutorials and critical appraisal tools are available [http://www.cebm.net/].

Centre for Evidence-Based Mental Health (CEBMH): CEBMH aims to 'promote the teaching and practice of evidence-based health care (EBHC) throughout the UK (with special emphasis on evidence-based mental health) and internationally. To develop, evaluate, and disseminate improved methods of using research in practice, and incorporate these in the teaching methods of the CEBMH' [http://cebmh.warne.ox.ac.uk/cebmh/index.html].

Centre for Reviews and Dissemination (CRD): CRD assembles and analyses data from multiple research studies to generate policy-relevant research. The Centre undertakes high-quality systematic reviews and associated economic evaluations, develops underpinning methods, and promotes and facilitates the use of research evidence in decision-making [https://www.york.ac.uk/crd/].

Cochrane CENTRAL: The largest collection of records of randomized controlled trials in the world [http://www.cochranelibrary.com/about/central-landing-page.html].

The Cochrane Collaboration: Their vision is 'that healthcare decision-making throughout the world will be informed by high-quality, timely research evidence'. They aim to help healthcare providers, policy-makers, patients, their advocates and carers, make well-informed decisions about healthcare, by preparing, updating, and promoting the accessibility of Cochrane Reviews [http://www.cochrane.org/].

Cochrane Evidence: In many languages [http://www.cochrane.org/search/site/?f[0]=im_field_stage%3A3&f[1]=im_field_stage%3A2&f[2]=im_field_stage%3A1].

****Cochrane Library:** Library for Cochrane Systematic Reviews, which are presented as full documents, summaries or plain language summaries [http://www.cochranelibrary.com/].

****Collaborating Centre for Social Care (NCCSC):** NCCSC develops guidance on social care for children and adults on behalf of the National Institute for Health and Care Excellence (NICE) [http://www.scie.org.uk/nccsc/index.asp].

Consolidated Standards of Reporting Trials (CONSORT): The CONSORT Statement (2010) is an evidence-based, minimum set of recommendations for reporting randomized controlled trials [http://www.consort-statement.org/].

Department of Health Essence of Care (2010): A set of established and refreshed benchmarks supporting front line care across care settings at a local level. It contains twelve benchmarks [https://www.gov.uk/government/publications/essence-of-care-2010].

Department of Health (UK) general site [http://www.dh.gov.uk/en/index.htm].

Department of Health (UK) policies [https://www.gov.uk/government/policies?organisations%5B%5D=department-of-health].

Department of Health (UK) statistics [https://www.gov.uk/government/statistics?keywords=&topics%5B%5D=all&departments%5B%5D=department-of-health&from_date=&to_date].

Enhancing the quality and transparency of health research (EQUATOR): The EQUATOR Network seeks to improve the reliability and value of published health research literature by offering reporting guidelines for the main study types [http://www.equator-network.org/].

Government (UK) social care policy [https://www.gov.uk/government/topics/social-care].

Health Knowledge: 'This learning resource is for anyone working in health, social care and well-being wherever they work or study. The resource allows you to access a broad range of learning materials for personal use or for teaching purposes in order to help everyone expand their **public health knowledge**.' The resources include a useful *Public Health Textbook* and various training courses and resources [https://www.healthknowledge.org.uk/].

King's Fund: The King's Fund is an independent charity working in England with the vision of achieving that the best possible health and care are available to all. The Fund offers a variety of publications and resources [http://www.kingsfund.org.uk/].

National Elf Service: A variety of resources for specific groups [https://www.nationalelfservice.net/], including:

Social care [https://www.nationalelfservice.net/about-social/]

Learning disabilities [https://www.nationalelfservice.net/learning-disabilities/]

Mental health [https://www.nationalelfservice.net/mental-health/]

National Guideline Clearinghouse: A US public resource for evidence-based clinical practice guidelines [https://www.guideline.gov/].

National Health Service Digital: Aims to provide national (UK) information, data, and IT systems for health and care services [https://digital.nhs.uk/article/190/Data-and-information].

**National Institute for Health and Care Excellence (NICE) 'NHS Evidence': This site offers NICE pathways, NICE guidance, standards and indicators, and evidence services, including the online British National Formulary (BNF) [https://www.evidence.nhs.uk/]. See below for more specific links.

National Institute for Health and Care Excellence (NICE) clinical knowledge summaries: Accessed alphabetically or by specialty [https://cks.nice.org.uk/#?char=A].

National Institute for Health and Care Excellence (NICE) pathways: Everything NICE says on a topic in an interactive flowchart [https://pathways.nice.org.uk/].

National Institute of Health Research (NIHR) evidence synthesis: [https://www.journalslibrary.nihr.ac.uk/search/#/?search=evidence%20

synthesis&sitekit=true&indexname=full-index&task=search&selected_ facets=].

Netting the Evidence: A custom search engine for all things related to evidence-based practice [https://cse.google.com/cse/home? cx=004326897958477606950:djcbsrxkatm].

PEDro – the Physiotherapy Evidence Database [https://www.pedro. org.au/].

Point of Care Foundation: Evidence and resources [https://www. pointofcarefoundation.org.uk/evidence-resources/].

PRISMA: An evidence-based minimum set of items for reporting in systematic reviews and meta-analyses. PRISMA focuses on the reporting of reviews evaluating randomized trials, but can also be used as a basis for reporting systematic reviews of other types of research, particularly evaluations of interventions [http://www.prisma-statement.org/].

Public Health England (PHE) data and analysis tools: An alphabetical listing of public health data and analysis tools from across Public Health England [https://www.gov.uk/guidance/phe-data-and-analysis-tools].

Public Health England (PHE) Public Health Outcomes framework: Find out about differences in life expectancy and healthy life expectancy between communities [http://www.phoutcomes.info/].

Scottish Intercollegiate Guidelines Network (SIGN): SIGN has a range of evidence-based guidelines [http://www.sign.ac.uk/guidelines/ index.html].

** Social Care Institute for Excellence (SCIE): SCIE aims to gather, analyse, and share knowledge about what works and translate that knowledge into practical resources, learning materials, and services, including training and consultancy. The notion of co-production is fundamental to what SCIE does. SCIE aims to co-produce its work with people who use services and carers [http://www.scie.org.uk/ and for a list of all their resources see: http://www.scie.org.uk/atoz/].

Social Care Institute for Excellence (SCIE) A–Z of research briefings [http://www.scie.org.uk/publications/briefings/index.asp**]**.

Social Care Institute for Excellence (SCIE) A–Z of research resources [http://www.scie.org.uk/atoz/?f_az_series_name=Research+ resource&page=1].

Social Care Online: A comprehensive, searchable database of information [http://www.scie-socialcareonline.org.uk/].

TripDatabase: A clinical search engine designed to allow users to quickly and easily find and use high-quality research evidence to support their practice and/or care [https://www.tripdatabase.com].

Appraisal tools/checklists

Appraisal of Guidelines for Research and Evaluation (AGREE): An instrument for evaluation of practice guideline development and the quality of reporting [http://www.agreetrust.org/].

**Critical Appraisal Skills Programme (CASP 2017): The CASP International Network is 'an international collaboration which supports the teaching and learning of critical appraisal skills'. A range of critical appraisal tools is available [http://www.caspinternational.org/].

DISCERN: A brief questionnaire that provides users with a valid and reliable way of assessing the quality of written information on treatment choices for a health problem. DISCERN can also be used by authors and publishers of information on treatment choices as a guide to the standard which users are entitled to expect [http://www.discern.org.uk/].

Glasgow University Institute of Health and Wellbeing: This site offers a variety of critical appraisal checklists [http://www.gla.ac.uk/research institutes/healthwellbeing/research/generalpractice/ebp/checklists/].

National Collaborating Centre for Methods and Tools (NCCMT): NCCMT (2015) *Appraising Qualitative, Quantitative, and Mixed Methods Studies Included in Mixed Studies Reviews: The MMAT*. Hamilton, ON: McMaster University (updated 20 July 2015) [available at: http://www.nccmt. ca/resources/search/232].

Scottish Intercollegiate Guidelines Network (SIGN): SIGN has a range of appraisal checklists [http://www.sign.ac.uk/methodology/checklists.html].

Students4BestEvidence: Contains blogs with appraised study examples [http://www.students4bestevidence.net/category/appraising-research/].

Useful video/audio

Ben Goldacre TED Talk (2011) *Battling bad science* [http://www.ted. com/talks/ben_goldacre_battling_bad_science].

Cochrane (2016) What are systematic reviews? [https://www.youtube.com/watch?v=egJlW4vkb1Y].

Cochrane podcasts: Deliver the latest Cochrane evidence in an easy to access audio format, allowing you to stay up to date on newly published reviews wherever you are. Each Cochrane podcast offers a short summary of a recent Cochrane review from the authors themselves. They have been recorded in more than 30 languages and are brief, allowing everyone from healthcare professionals to patients and families to hear the latest Cochrane evidence in under five minutes. Browse the podcasts or use the search box to look for something specific [http://www.cochrane.org/multimedia/podcasts/].

McCormack, J. (2013) Viva La Evidence!: A parody of Coldplay's Viva La Vida, this is a song all about evidence-based healthcare – a little bit about the history of evidence and then the key principles [https://www.youtube.com/watch?v=QUW0Q8tXVUc].

McMasters University online tutorials [http://hsl.mcmaster.libguides.com/tutorials].

National Institute for Health and Care Excellence (NICE) slides of clinical knowledge summaries [https://cks.nice.org.uk/slides].

Research in Practice for Adults (RIPFA): RIPFA has produced a short film 'What is evidence informed practice?' that shows how they use evidence to support social work practice with adults and their families [https://www.ripfa.org.uk/latest-news/what-is-evidence-informed-practice/].

Social Care TV channel: The channel includes a collection of video resources [http://www.scie.org.uk/socialcaretv/index.asp].

Professional bodies

Health and Care Professions Council (HCPC): HCPC is a regulator set up to protect the public. To do this, they keep a Register of Health and Care Professionals who meet the standards for training, professional skills, behaviour, and health. They regulate the following professions: arts therapists, biomedical scientists, chiropodists/podiatrists, clinical scientists, dietitians, hearing aid dispensers, occupational therapists, operating department practitioners, orthoptists, paramedics, physiotherapists, practitioner psychologists, prosthetists/orthotists, radiographers, social workers in England, and speech and language therapists [http://www.hcpc-uk.org/].

Nursing and Midwifery Council (NMC): The NMC is the regulatory body for nurses and midwives in England, Wales, Scotland, and Northern Ireland. They exist to protect the public. They also set standards of education, training, conduct, and performance so that nurses and midwives can deliver high-quality healthcare throughout their careers. They make sure that nurses and midwives keep their skills and knowledge up to date and uphold professional standards. They also have clear and transparent processes to investigate nurses and midwives who fall short of the standards and maintain a register of nurses and midwives allowed to practise in the UK [https://www.nmc.org.uk/].

Public Health England: Population screening pathways [https://www.gov.uk/government/collections/nhs-population-screening-care-pathways].

Useful social media sites and information

The remit of this book does not allow a full overview of social media. However, it is a medium that can be used by professionals and patients/clients to share evidence or information, to network, and to get support or advice. This can be via many formats including:

• Social networking (e.g. Facebook, Twitter)
• Media (e.g.YouTube, Flickr)
• Blogs (e.g. Tumblr, WordPress)

Using social media professionally

You need to be aware of your **professional responsibilities**. For in the UK, see:

NMC (2016) Guidance on using social media responsibly [https://www.nmc.org.uk/standards/guidance/social-media-guidance/].

Health and Care Professions Council (no date) Use of social networking sites [http://www.hpc-uk.org/registrants/standards/socialnetworking/].

Helpful sites for learning about social media use

• **Facebook** [https://www.facebook.com/help/104002523024878]
• **Twitter** [https://support.twitter.com/]
• **Blogs** [https://www.bloggingbasics101.com/how-do-i-start-a-blog/]
• **Skills for Health: The social media toolkit for healthcare** [http://www.skillsforhealth.org.uk/socialtoolkit].
• **We Communities – Twitterversity:** How to use Twitter professionally [http://www.wecommunities.org/resources/twitterversity].

Relevant articles

Huby, K. and Smith, J. (2016) Relevance of social media to nurses and healthcare: 'to tweet or not to tweet', *Evidence-Based Nursing*, 19 (4): 105–106.

Moorley, C. and Chinn, T. (2015) Using social media for continuous professional development, *Journal of Advanced Nursing*, 71 (4): 713–717.

Sinclair, W., McLoughlin, M. and Warne, T. (2015) To twitter to woo: harnessing the power of social media (SoMe) in nurse education to enhance the student's experience, *Nurse Education in Practice*, 15 (6): 507–511.

Facebook

* Cochrane [https://www.facebook.com/TheCochraneLibrary/]
* Students4Best Evidence [https://www.facebook.com/Students4BE]

Twitter

Consider setting up a professional Twitter account. See Signing up with Twitter *[https://support.twitter.com/articles/100990].*

The following Twitter handles are used for different professions:

@WeNurses for more General/Adult nursing issues
@WeAHP for Allied Health Professions
@WeMHNurse for Mental Health Nurses
@WeCYP for Children and Young People Nurses
@WeLDnurses for Learning Disability Nurse
@WeGPNs for General Practice Nurses
@WeHVs for Health Visitors
@WeParamedics for Paramedics and in Australia @WePharmerOz
@WePharmacists for Pharmacists
@WeSchoolNurses for School Nurses
@WeMidwives for Midwives
@WeDistrictNurse for District Nurses
@WeDocs for Doctors

For **Twitter Chat** information, see http://www.wecommunities.org/tweet-chats/chat-calendar. Remember to use the relevant hashtags and you may find **Tweetdeck** useful to help you in a Twitter chat [https://tweetdeck.twitter.com].

See the following sites to find out about the Cochrane Twitter accounts:

Cochrane Library of systematic reviews account @CochraneLibrary
Cochrane 'Critical appraisal Twitter Session' (#WeCats) [http://www.
   casp-uk.net/wecats] (#WeCats)
http://uk.cochrane.org/evidence-everyday-nursing
http://uk.cochrane.org/evidence-everyday-allied-health
http://uk.cochrane.org/evidence-everyday-health-choices
http://uk.cochrane.org/evidence-everyday-midwifery
http://uk.cochrane.org/students-4-best-evidence

Blogs

http://uk.cochrane.org/understanding-evidence
http://www.evidentlycochrane.net/
http://www.students4bestevidence.net/

References

Abou-Setta, A.M., Jeyaraman, M.M., Attia, A., Al-Inany, H.G., Ferri, M., Ansari, M.T. et al. (2016) Methods for developing evidence reviews in short periods of time: a scoping review, *PLoS ONE*, 11 (12): e0165903 [available at: http://journals.plos. org/plosone/article?id=10.1371/journal.pone.0165903].

Albrecht, L., Archibald, M., Snelgrove-Clarke, E. and Scott, S.D. (2016) Systematic review of knowledge translation strategies to promote research uptake in child health settings, *Journal of Pediatric Nursing*, 31 (3): 235–254.

Allen, N.E., Beral, V., Casabonne, D., Kan, S.-W., Reeves, G.K., Brown, A. et al. (2009) Moderate alcohol intake and cancer incidence in women, *Journal of the National Cancer Institute*, 101 (5): 296–305.

Appleby, L., Shaw, J., Amos, T., McDonnell, R., Harris, C., McCann, K. et al. (1999) Suicide within 12 months of contact with mental health services: national clinical survey, *British Medical Journal*, 318 (7193): 1235–1239.

Aromataris, E. and Riitano, D. (2014) Constructing a search strategy and searching for evidence: a guide to the literature search for a systematic review, *American Journal of Nursing*, 114 (5): 49–56.

Aveyard, H. (2010) *Doing a Literature Review in Health and Social Care*. Maidenhead: Open University Press.

Aveyard, H. (2014) *Doing a Literature Review in Health and Social Care*, 2nd edn. Maidenhead: Open University Press.

Aveyard, H., Sharp, P. and Woolliams, M. (2015) *A Beginner's Guide to Critical Thinking and Writing in Health and Social Care*. Maidenhead: Open University Press.

Aveyard, P.N., Lewis, A., Tearne, S., Hood, K., Christian-Brown, A., Adab, P. et al. (2016) Screening and brief intervention for obesity in primary care: a parallel two arm randomized control trial, *Lancet*, 388 (10059): 2492–2500.

Baker, R., Camosso-Stefinovic, J., Gillies, C., Shaw, J.E., Cheater, F., Flottrop, S. et al. (2015) Tailored interventions to address determinants of practice, *Cochrane Database of Systematic Reviews*, 4: CD005470 [available at: http://onlinelibrary. wiley.com/doi/10.1002/14651858.CD005470.pub3/full].

Barlow, J. (2016) *Effects of Parenting Programmes: a review of 6 Campbell systematic reviews*, Campbell Policy Brief #1, The Campbell Collaboration.

Beauchamp, T. and Childress, J.F. (2013) *Principles of Biomedical Ethics*, 7th edn. Oxford: Oxford University Press.

Benner, P. (1984) *From Novice to Expert*. New York: Addison-Wesley.

Benner, P. and Tanner, C.A. (1987) Clinical judgement: how expert nurses use intuition, *American Journal of Nursing*, 87 (1): 23–31.

Bergs, J., Lambrechts, F., Simons, P., Vlayen, A., Marneffe, W., Hellings, J. et al. (2015) Barriers and facilitators related to the implementation of surgical safety checklists: a systematic review of the qualitative evidence, *BMJ Quality and Safety*, 24 (12): 776–786.

BestBets (n.d.) *Best evidence topics* [available at: http://bestbets.org/index.php; accessed 8 May 2017].

Birnbaum, R. and Saini, M. (2012) A qualitative synthesis of children's participation in custody disputes, *Research on Social Work Practice*, 22 (4): 400–409.

Booth, A. (2016) Searching for qualitative research for inclusion in systematic reviews: a structured methodological review, *Systematic Reviews*, 5: 74 [available at: https://systematicreviewsjournal.biomedcentral.com/articles/10.1186/s13643-016-0249-x?].

Bradshaw, A. and Price, L. (2006) Rectal suppositories insertion: the reliability of the evidence as a basis for nursing practice, *Journal of Clinical Nursing*, 16 (1): 98–103.

Bramer, W.M., Giustini, D. and Kramer, B.M. (2016) Comparing the coverage, recall, and precision of searches for 120 systematic reviews in Embase, MEDLINE, and Google Scholar: a prospective study, *Systematic Reviews*, 5: 39 [available at: https://systematicreviewsjournal.biomedcentral.com/articles/10.1186/s13643-016-0215-7].

Briscoe, S. and Cooper, C. (2014) The British Nursing Index and CINAHL: a comparison of journal title coverage and the implications for information professionals, *Health Information and Libraries Journal*, 31 (3): 195–203.

Buchanan, H., Jelsma, J. and Siegfried, N. (2015) Measuring evidence-based practice knowledge and skills in occupational therapy – a brief instrument, *BMC Medical Education*, 15 (1): 191.

Bulman, C., Forde-Johnson, C., Griffiths, A., Hallsworth, S., Kerry, A., Khan, S. et al. (2016) The development of peer reflective supervision amongst nurse educator colleagues: an action research project, *Nurse Education Today*, 45: 148–155.

Caddick, N., Varela-Mato, V., Nimmo, M.A., Clemes, S., Yates, T. and King, J.A. (2017) Understanding the health of lorry drivers in context: a critical discourse analysis, *Health*, 21 (1): 38–56.

Care Quality Commission (2016) *Health and Social Care Act 2008 (Regulated Activities) Regulations 2014: Regulation 20: Duty of Candour* [available at: http://www.cqc.org.uk/content/regulation-20-duty-candour#full-regulation].

CASP International (2017) *Critical Appraisal Skills Programme* (CASP) [available at: http://www.casp-uk.net/casp-international].

Castro, E.M., Van Regenmortel, T., Vanhaecht, K., Sermeus, W. and Van Hecke, A. (2016) Patient empowerment, patient participation and patient-centeredness in hospital care: a concept analysis based on a literature review, *Patient Education and Counseling*, 99 (12): 1923–1939.

Cochrane Community (2016) *Cochrane strategy to 2020* [available at: http://community.cochrane.org/organizational-info/resources/strategy-2020].CONSORT (2010) *The CONSORT statement* [available at: http://www.consort-statement.org/].

Corbett, A., Achterberg, W., Husebo, B., Lobbezoo, F., de Vet, H., Kunz, M. et al. (2014) An international road map to improve pain assessment in people with impaired cognition: the development of the Pain Assessment in Impaired Cognition (PAIC) meta-tool, *BMC Neurology*, 14: 229 [available at: https://bmcneurol.biomedcentral.com/articles/10.1186/s12883-014-0229-5].

Cottrell, S. (2017) *Critical Thinking Skills*, 3rd edn. Basingstoke: Palgrave Macmillan.

Crabtree, J.L., Justiss, M. and Swinehart, S. (2012) Occupational therapy master-level students' evidence-based practice knowledge and skills before and after fieldwork, *Occupational Therapy in Health Care*, 26 (2/3): 138–149.

Crowe, M. and Sheppard, I. (2011) A review of critical appraisal tools show they lack rigor: alternative tool structure is proposed, *Journal of Clinical Epidemiology*, 64 (1): 79–89.

Cumming, E. and Henry, W.E. (1961) *Growing Old: The process of disengagement.* New York: Basic Books.

Dadkhah, M., Jazi, M.D. and Pacukaj, S. (2015) Fake conferences for earning real money, *Mediterranean Journal of Social Sciences*, 6 (2): 11–12.

Darbyshire, P., McKenna, L., Lee, S.F. and East, C.E. (2016) Taking a stand against predatory publishers, *Journal of Advanced Nursing* [doi: 10.1111/jan.13004].

Dawes, M., Summerskill, W. and Glasziou, P. (2005) Sicily statement on evidence-based practice, *BMC Medical Education*, 5: 1 [available at: https://bmcmededuc.biomedcentral.com/articles/10.1186/1472-6920-5-1].

Department of Constitutional Affairs (2005) *Mental Capacity Act: Code of practice.* London: The Stationery Office [available at: http://www.legislation.gov.uk/ukpga/2005/9/contents].

Department of Health (2010) *Essence of Care.* London: Department of Health [available at: https://www.gov.uk/government/publications/essence-of-care-2010].

Department of Health (2011) *Clinical Governance Guidance.* London: Department of Health [available at: https://www.gov.uk/government/news/clinical-governance-guidance].

Dignity in Care (2014) Challenging poor practice – training module [available at: http://www.dignityincare.org.uk/Resources/Type/Challenging-Poor-Practice-Training-module/].

Dogherty, E.J., Harrison, M.B., Graham, I.D., Vandyk, A.D. and Keeping-Burke, L. (2013) Turning knowledge into action at the point-of-care: the collective experience of nurses facilitating the implementation of evidence-based practice, *Worldviews on Evidence-Based Nursing*, 10 (3): 129–139.

Doll, R. and Hill, A.B. (1954) The mortality of doctors in relation to their smoking habits, *British Medical Journal*, 228: 1451–1455.

Douw, G., Schoonhoven, L., Holwerda, T., van Zanten, A.R., van Achterberg, T. and van der Hoeven, J.G. (2015) Nurses' worry or concern and early recognition of deteriorating patients on general wards in acute care hospitals: a systematic review, *Critical Care*, 19: 230 [available at: https://ccforum.biomedcentral.com/articles/10.1186/s13054-015-0950-5].

Downes, M.J., Brennan, M.L., Williams, H.C. and Dean, R.S. (2016) Development of a critical appraisal tool to assess the quality of cross-sectional studies (AXIS), *BMJ Open*, 6 (12): e011458 [available at: http://eprints.nottingham.ac.uk/39316/1/BMJ%20Open-2016-Downes-.pdf].

Drummond, M. (2016) Clinical guidelines: a NICE way to introduce cost-effectiveness considerations?, *Value in Health*, 19 (5): 525–530.

Dunn, P. (1997) James Lind (1716–94) of Edinburgh and the treatment of scurvy, *Archives of Diseases in Childhood: Fetal and Neonatal Edition*, 76 (1): F64–F65.

Ejemot-Nwadiaro, R.I., Ehiri, J.E., Arikpo, D., Meremikwu, M.M. and Critchley, J.A. (2015) Hand washing promotion for preventing diarrhoea, *Cochrane Database of Systematic Reviews*, 9: CD004265 [available at: http://onlinelibrary.wiley.com/doi/10.1002/14651858.CD004265.pub3/full].

Farley, A.C., Hajek, P., Lycett, D. and Aveyard, P. (2012) Interventions for preventing weight gain after smoking cessation, *Cochrane Database of Systematic Reviews*, 1: CD006219 [available at: http://onlinelibrary.wiley.com/doi/10.1002/14651858.CD006219.pub3/full].

Featherstone, R.M., Dryden, D.M., Foisy, M., Guise, J.M., Mitchell, M.D., Paynter, R.A. et al. (2015) Advancing knowledge of rapid reviews: an analysis of results, conclusions and recommendations from published review articles examining rapid reviews, *Systematic Reviews*, 4: 50 [available at: https://systematicreviewsjournal.biomedcentral.com/articles/10.1186/s13643-015-0040-4].

Ferguson, C., DiGiacomo, M., Gholizadeh, L., Ferguson, L.E. and Hickman, L.D. (2017) The integration and evaluation of a social-media facilitated journal club to enhance the student learning experience of evidence-based practice: a case study, *Nurse Education Today*, 48: 123–128.

Fineout-Overholt, E. and Johnston, L. (2005) Teaching evidence-based practice: asking searchable, answerable clinical questions, *Worldviews on Evidence-Based Nursing*, 2 (3): 157–160.

Fineout-Overholt, E. and Melnyk, B.M. (2006) *Organizational Culture and Readiness for System-Wide Implementation of EBP (OCRSIEP) Scale.* Gilbert, AZ: ARCC Publishing.

Finfgeld-Connett, D. and Johnson, E.D. (2013) Literature search strategies for conducting knowledge-building and theory-generating qualitative systematic reviews, *Journal of Advanced Nursing*, 69 (1): 194–204.

Fisher, B., Anderson, S., Bryant, J., Margolese, R.G., Deutsch, M., Fisher, E.R. et al. (2002) Twenty-year follow-up of a randomized trial comparing total mastectomy, lumpectomy, and lumpectomy plus irradiation for the treatment of invasive breast cancer, *New England Journal of Medicine*, 347 (16): 1233–1241.

Flodgren, G., Rachas, A., Farmer, A.J., Inzitari, M. and Shepperd, S. (2015) Interactive telemedicine: effects on professional practice and health care outcomes, *Cochrane Database of Systematic Reviews*, 9: CD002098 [available at: http://onlinelibrary.wiley.com/store/10.1002/14651858.CD002098.pub2/asset/CD002098.pdf?v=1&t=j3twktjr&s=52dc518d3644fc9d75bf11a9eec2818ef69be67a].

Francis, R. (2013) *Report of the Mid Staffordshire NHS Foundation Trust Public Enquiry: Final Report.* London: The Stationery Office [available at: http://webarchive.nationalarchives.gov.uk/20150407084003/http://www.midstaffspublicinquiry.com/report].

Fraser, A.G. and Dunstan, F.D. (2010) On the impossibility of being expert, *British Medical Journal*, 341: c6815.

Friesen-Storms, J., Moser, A., Van der Loo, S., Beurskens, A. and Bours, G. (2014) Systematic implementation of evidence-based practice in a clinical nursing setting: a participatory action research project, *Journal of Clinical Nursing*, 24 (1/2): 57–68.

Fulford, K.W.M., Peile, E. and Carroll, H. (2012) *Essential Values-Based Practice: Clinical stories linking science with people.* Cambridge: Cambridge University Press.

Gerrish, K., McDonnell, A.M., Nolan, M., Guillaume, L., Kirshbaum, M. and Tod, A. (2011) The role of advanced practice nurses in knowledge brokering as a means of promoting evidence-based practice among clinical nurses, *Journal of Advanced Nursing,* 67 (9): 2004–2014.

Giles, T., de Lacey, S. and Muir-Cochrane, E. (2016) Factors influencing decision making around family presence during resuscitation: a grounded theory study, *Journal of Advanced Nursing,* 72 (11): 2706–2717.

Glegg, S.M., Livingstone, R. and Montgomery, I. (2016) Facilitating interprofessional evidence-based practice in paediatric rehabilitation: development, implementation and evaluation of an online toolkit for health professionals, *Disability and Rehabilitation,* 38 (4): 391–399.

Goldacre, B. (2008) *Bad Science.* London: HarperCollins.

Gottwald, M. and Lansdown, G. (2014) *Clinical Governance.* Maidenhead: Open University Press.

Graff, C. (2016) Mixed methods research, in H.R. Hall and L.A. Roussel (eds) *Evidence-based Practice: An integrative approach to research administration and practice.* Burlington, MA: Jones & Bartlett.

Graham, C., West, W., Bourdon, J., Ilge, K.J. and Seward, H.E. (2016) Employment interventions for return to work in working aged adults following traumatic brain injury (TBI): A systematic review, *Campbell Systematic Reviews,* 2016: 6 [available at: https://www.campbellcollaboration.org/media/k2/attachments/Graham_Employment_Interventions_Review.pdf].

Gray, J.K. and Grove, S.K. (2016) Critical appraisal of nursing studies, in J.K. Gray, S.K. Grove and S. Sutherland, *The Practice of Nursing Research: Appraisal, synthesis and generation of evidence,* 8th edn. St. Louis, MO: Saunders.

Gray, M., Joy, E., Plath, D. and Webb, S.A. (2014) Opinions about evidence: a study of social workers' attitudes towards evidence-based practice, *Journal of Social Work,* 14 (1): 23–40.

Gray, M., Sharland, E., Heinsch, M. and Schubert, L. (2015) Connecting research to action: perspectives on research utilization, *British Journal of Social Work,* 45 (7): 1952–1967.

Greenhalgh, T. (2014) *How to Read a Paper: The basics of evidence-based medicine,* 5th edn. Chichester: Wiley-Blackwell/BMJ Books.

Greenway, K. (2014) Rituals in nursing: intramuscular injections, *Journal of Clinical Nursing,* 25 (4): 264–265.

Griffiths, R. (2017) Assessing Gillick competence, *British Journal of Midwifery,* 25 (4): 264.

Harvey, G. and Kitson, A. (2015a) Translating evidence into healthcare policy and practice: single versus multi-faceted implementation strategies – is there a simple answer to a complex question?, *International Journal of Health Policy and Management,* 4 (3): 123–126.

Harvey, G. and Kitson, A. (2015b) *Implementing Evidence-based Practice in Healthcare: A facilitation guide.* Abingdon: Routledge.

Harvey, G. and Kitson, A. (2016) PARIHS revisited: from heuristic to integrated framework for the successful implementation of knowledge into practice, *Implementation Science*, 11 (1): 33.

Hastie, R. and Dawes, R.M. (2010) *Rational Choice in an Uncertain World*, 2nd edn. Thousand Oaks, CA: Sage.

Health and Care Professions Council (HCPC) (2016) *Standards of Conduct, Performance and Ethics* [available at: http://www.hpc-uk.org/aboutregistration/standards/].

Health and Care Professions Council (HCPC) (2017) *Raising and escalating concerns in the workplace* [available at: http://www.hpc-uk.org/registrants/raising-concerns/].

Health Foundation, The (2014) *Ideas into Action: Person-centred care in practice – what to consider when implementing shared decision making and self-management support*. London: The Health Foundation [available at: http://www.health.org.uk/sites/health/files/IdeasIntoActionPersonCentredCareInPractice.pdf].

Hecht, L., Buhse, S. and Meyer, G. (2016) Effectiveness of training in evidence-based medicine skills for healthcare professionals: a systematic review, *BMC Medical Education*, 16 (1): 103.

Heneghan, C., Spencer, E.A., Bobrovitz, N., Collins, D.R.J., Nunan, D., Plüddemann, A. et al. (2016) Lack of evidence for interventions offered in UK fertility centres. *British Medical Journal*, 355: i6295.

Heydari, A., Mazlom, S.R., Ranjbar, H. and Scurlock-Evans, L. (2014). A study of Iranian nurses' and midwives' knowledge, attitudes, and implementation of evidence-based practice: the time for change has arrived, *Worldviews on Evidence-Based Nursing*, 11 (5): 325–331.

Higgins, J.P.T. and Altman, D.G. (2008) Assessing risk of bias in included studies, in J.P.T. Higgins and S. Green (eds) *Cochrane Handbook for Systematic Reviews of Interventions*. Chichester: Wiley.

Horsley, T., Dingwall, O. and Sampson, M. (2011a) Checking reference lists to find additional studies for systematic reviews, *Cochrane Database of Systematic Reviews*, 8: MR000026 [available at: http://onlinelibrary.wiley.com/doi/10.1002/14651858.MR000026.pub2/full].

Howe, W. (2001/2010) *Evaluating quality* [available at: http://www.walthowe.com/navnet/quality.html].

Huby, K. and Smith, J. (2016) Relevance of social media to nurses and healthcare: 'to tweet or not to tweet', *Evidence-Based Nursing*, 19 (4): 105–106.

Ilic, D., Nordin, R.B., Glasziou, P., Tilson, J.K. and Villanueva, E. (2014) Development and validation of the ACE tool: assessing medical trainees' competency in evidence based medicine, *BMC Medical Education*, 14 (1): 114.

Jefferson, T., Del Mar, C.B., Dooley, L., Ferroni, E., Al-Ansary, L.A., Bawazeer, G.A. et al. (2011) Physical interventions to interrupt or reduce the spread of respiratory viruses, *Cochrane Database of Systematic Reviews*, 7: CD006207 [available at: http://onlinelibrary.wiley.com/doi/10.1002/14651858.CD006207.pub4/full].

Jones, R., Kelsey, J., Nelmes, P., Chinn, N., Chinn, T. and Proctor-Childs, T. (2016). Introducing Twitter as an assessed component of the undergraduate nursing curriculum: case study, *Journal of Advanced Nursing*, 72 (7): 1638–1653.

Jun, J., Kovner, C.T. and Stimpfel, A.W. (2016) Barriers and facilitators of nurses' use of clinical practice guidelines: an integrative review, *International Journal of Nursing Studies*, 60: 54–68.

Kailasam, V.K. and Samuels, E. (2015) Can social media help mental health practitioners prevent suicides? Anecdotal evidence suggests that analyzing Facebook posts can lead to earlier intervention, *Current Psychiatry*, 14 (2): 37–39, 51.

Kajermo, K.N., Boström, A.M., Thompson, D.S., Hutchinson, A.M., Estabrooks, C.A. and Wallin, L. (2010) The BARRIERS scale – the barriers to research utilization scale: a systematic review, *Implementation Science*, 5: 32 [available at: http://www.implementationscience.com/content/5/1/32].

Katrak, P., Blalocerkowski, A.E., Massy-Westropp, N., Saravana Kumar, V.S. and Grimmer, K.A. (2004) A systematic review of the content of critical appraisal tools, *BMC Medical Research Methodology*, 4: 22 [available at: http://www.biomedcentral.com/content/pdf/1471-2288-4-22.pdf].

Kim, S.C., Brown, C.E., Ecoff, L., Davidson, J.E., Gallo, A.M., Klimpel, K. et al. (2013) Regional evidence-based practice fellowship program: impact on evidence-based practice implementation and barriers, *Clinical Nursing Research*, 22 (1): 51–69.

Kitchens, B., Harle, C.A. and Li, S. (2014) Quality of health-related online search results, *Decision Support Systems*, 57: 454–462.

Kmietowicz, Z. (2012) University College London issues new research standards but says it won't investigate Wakefield, *British Medical Journal*, 345: e6220.

Knipschild, P. (1994) Systematic reviews: some examples, *British Medical Journal*, 309: 719.

Kredo, T., Bernhardsson, S., Machingaidze, S., Young, T., Louw, Q., Ochodo, E. et al. (2016) Guide to clinical practice guidelines: the current state of play, *International Journal for Quality in Health Care*, 28 (1): 122–128.

Kumar, A. and Maskara, S. (2015) Coping up with information overload in the medical profession, *Journal of Biosciences and Medicines*, 3: 124–127.

Kyriakoulis, K., Patelarou, A., Laliotis, A., Wan, A.C., Matalliotakis, M., Tsiou, C. et al. (2016) Educational strategies for teaching evidence based practice to undergraduate students: systematic review, *Journal of Educational Evaluation for Health Professionals*, 13: 34.

Launey, E., Cohen, J.F., Morfouace, M., Gras-Le Guen, C., Ravaud, P. and Chalumeau, M. (2016) Inadequate critical appraisal of studies in systematic reviews of time to diagnosis, *Journal of Clinical Epidemiology*, 78: 43–51.

Leach, M.J. and Gillham, D. (2008) Evaluation of the Evidence-Based practice Attitude and utilization SurvEy for complementary and alternative medicine practitioners, *Journal of Evaluation in Clinical Practice*, 14 (5): 792–798.

Leach, M.J., Hofmeyer, A. and Bobridge, A. (2016) The impact of research education on student nurse attitude, skill and uptake of evidence-based practice: a descriptive longitudinal survey, *Journal of Clinical Nursing*, 25 (1/2): 194–203.

Légaré, F., Stacey, D., Turcotte, S., Cossi, M., Kryworuchko, J., Graham, I.D. et al. (2014) Interventions for improving the adoption of shared decision making by healthcare professionals, *Cochrane Database of Systematic Reviews*, 9: CD006732 [available at: http://onlinelibrary.wiley.com/doi/10.1002/14651858.CD006732.pub3/full].

Lessen, R. and Kavanagh, K. (2015) Position of the Academy of Nutrition and Dietetics: promoting and supporting breastfeeding, *Journal of the Academy of Nutrition and Dietetics*, 115 (3): 444–449.

Leung, K., Trevena, L. and Waters, D. (2016) Development of a competency framework for evidence-based practice in nursing, *Nurse Education Today*, 39: 189–196.

Lincoln, Y.S. and Guba, E.G. (1985) *Naturalistic Inquiry*. Beverly Hills, CA: Sage.

Llasus, L., Angosta, A.D. and Clark, M. (2014) Graduating baccalaureate students' evidence-based practice knowledge, readiness, and implementation, *Journal of Nursing Education*, 53 (9): S82–S89.

Magrunder, K.M., York, J.A., Knapp, R.G., Yeager, D.E., Marshall, E. and DeSantis, M. (2016) RCT evaluating provider outcomes by suicide prevention training modality: in-person vs. e-learning, *Journal of Mental Health Training, Education and Practice*, 10 (4): 207–217.

Mallion, J. and Brooke, J. (2016) Community-and hospital-based nurses' implementation of evidence-based practice: are there any differences?, *British Journal of Community Nursing*, 21 (3): 148–154.

Maltby, H.J., de Vries-Erich, J.M. and Lund, K. (2016) Being the stranger: comparing study abroad experiences of nursing students in low and high income countries through hermeneutical phenomenology, *Nurse Education Today*, 45: 114–119.

Manaseki-Holland, S., Bavuusuren, B., Bayandarj, T., Sprachman, S. and Marshall, T. (2010) Effects of traditional swaddling on development: a randomised controlled trial, *Paediatrics*, 126 (6): e1485–e1492.

Massey, D., Chaboyer, W. and Anderson, V. (2017) What factors influence ward nurses' recognition of and response to patient deterioration? An integrative review of the literature, *Nursing Open*, 4 (1): 6–23 [available at: https://www.ncbi.nlm.nih.gov/pmc/articles/PMC5221430/pdf/NOP2-4-6.pdf].

McArthur, A., Klugarova, J., Yan, H. and Florescu, S. (2015) Innovations in the systematic review of text and opinion, *International Journal of Evidence-Based Healthcare*, 13: 188–195 [see also: http://joannabriggs.org/assets/docs/critical-appraisal-tools/JBI_Critical_Appraisal-Checklist_for_Text_and_Opinion.pdf].

McCambridge, J., Witton, J. and Elbourne, D.R. (2014) Systematic review of the Hawthorne effect: new concepts are needed to study research participation effects, *Journal of Clinical Epidemiology*, 67 (3): 267–277.

McGinn, T., Taylor, B., McColgan, M. and McQuilkan, J. (2016) Social work literature searching: current issues with databases and online search engines, *Research on Social Work Practice*, 26 (3): 266–277.

McGraughey, J., Alderdice, F., Fowler, R., Kapila, A., Mayhew, A. and Moutray, M. (2009) Outreach and early warning systems for the prevention of intensive care admission and death of critically ill adult patients on general hospital wards, *Cochrane Database of Systematic Reviews*, 3: CD005529 [available at: http://onlinelibrary.wiley.com/doi/10.1002/14651858.CD005529.pub2/full].

McHale, P., Keenan, A. and Ghebrehewet, S. (2016) Reasons for measles cases not being vaccinated with MMR: investigation into parents' and carers' views following a large measles outbreak, *Epidemiology and Infection*, 144 (4): 870–875.

McKee, R. (2013) Ethical issues in using social media for health and health care research, *Health Policy*, 110 (2): 298–301.

McKeever, S., Kinney, S., Lima, S. and Newall, F. (2016) Creating a journal club competition improves paediatric nurses' participation and engagement, *Nurse Education Today*, 37: 173–177.

Mckew, M. (2017) Ward patients urged to get up, dressed and mobile, *Nursing Standard*, 31 (24): 10.

Mellis, C. (2015) Measles-mumps-rubella vaccine does not cause autism, *Journal of Paediatric and Child Health*, 51 (8): 838.

Melnyk, B.M. (2016a) Level of evidence plus critical appraisal of its quality yields confidence to implement evidence based practice changes, *Worldviews on Evidence-Based Nursing*, 13 (5): 332–339.

Melnyk, B.M. (2016b) Culture eats strategy every time: what works in building and sustaining an evidence-based practice culture in healthcare systems, *Worldviews on Evidence-Based Nursing*, 13 (2): 99–101.

Melnyk, B.M. and Fineout-Overholt, E. (2014) *Evidence-based Practice in Nursing and Healthcare: A guide to best practice*, 3rd edn. Philadelphia, PA: Wolters Kluwer.

Melnyk, B.M., Fineout-Overholt, E., Giggleman, M. and Choy, K. (2017) A test of the ARCC© model improves implementation of evidence-based practice, healthcare culture, and patient outcomes, *Worldviews on Evidence-Based Nursing*, 14 (1): 5–9.

Melnyk, B.M., Fineout-Overholt, E., Stillwell, B. and Williamson, K.M. (2009) Evidence-based practice. Step by step: igniting a spirit of inquiry, *American Journal of Nursing*, 109 (11): 49–52.

Melnyk, B.M., Fineout-Overholt, E., Stillwell, S.B. and Williamson, K.M. (2010) Evidence-based practice. Step by step: the seven steps of evidence-based practice, *American Journal of Nursing*, 110 (1): 51–53.

Melnyk, B.M., Gallagher-Ford, L. and Fineout-Overholt, E. (2016a) *Implementing the Evidence-Based Practice (EBP) Competencies in Healthcare: A practical guide for improving quality, safety, and outcomes*. Indianapolis, IN: Sigma Theta Tau International.

Melnyk, B.M., Gallagher-Ford, L., Long, L.E. and Fineout-Overholt, E. (2014) The establishment of evidence-based practice competencies for practicing registered nurses and advanced practice nurses in real-world clinical settings: proficiencies to improve healthcare quality, reliability, patient outcomes, and costs, *Worldviews on Evidence-Based Nursing*, 11 (1): 5–15.

Melnyk, B.M., Gallagher-Ford, L., Thomas, B.K., Troseth, M., Wyngarden, K. and Szalacha, L. (2016b) A study of chief nurse executives indicates low prioritization of evidence-based practice and shortcomings in hospital performance metrics across the United States, *Worldviews on Evidence-Based Nursing*, 13 (1): 6–14.

Miles, A. and Loughlin, M. (2011) Models in the balance: evidence-based medicine versus evidence-informed individualized care, *Journal of Evaluation in Clinical Practice*, 17 (4): 531–536.

Moher, D., Liberati, A., Tetzlaff, J., Altman, D.G. and Prisma Group (2009) Preferred reporting items for systematic reviews and meta-analyses: the PRISMA statement, *PLoS Medicine*, 6 (7): e1000097 [available at: http://journals.plos.org/plosmedicine/article?id=10.1371/journal.pmed.1000097].

Moorley, C. and Chinn, T. (2015) Using social media for continuous professional development, *Journal of Advanced Nursing*, 71 (4): 713–717.

Moule, P. (2015) *Making Sense of Research in Nursing, Health and Social Care.* London: Sage.

Murthy, L., Shepperd, S., Clarke, M.J., Garner, S.E., Lavis, J.N., Perrier, L. et al. (2012) Interventions to improve the use of systematic reviews in decision-making by health system managers, policy makers and clinicians, *Cochrane Database of Systematic Reviews*, 9: CD009401 [available at: http://onlinelibrary.wiley.com/doi/10.1002/14651858.CD009401.pub2/full].

Nagayama, H., Tomori, K., Ohno, K., Takahashi, K. and Yamauchi, K. (2015) Cost-effectiveness of occupational therapy in older people: systematic review of randomized controlled trials, *Occupational Therapy International*, 23 (2): 103–120.

National Collaborating Centre for Methods and Tools (NCCMT) (2015) *Appraising Qualitative, Quantitative, and Mixed Methods Studies Included in Mixed Studies Reviews: The MMAT.* Hamilton, ON: McMaster University (updated 20 July 2015) [available at: http://www.nccmt.ca/resources/search/232].

National Institute for Health Research (2014) Guidance on the use of social media to actively involve people in research [available at: http://www.invo.org.uk/wp-content/uploads/2014/11/9982-Social-Media-Guide-WEB.pdf].

Nevo, I. and Slonim-Nevo, V. (2011) The myth of evidence-based practice: towards evidence-informed practice, *British Journal of Social Work*, 41 (6): 1176–1197.

NHS England (2014) *Sign up to Safety* [available at: https://www.england.nhs.uk/signuptosafety/about/].

NHS England (2017) *Shared Decision Making* [available at: https://www.england.nhs.uk/ourwork/pe/sdm/].

NICE (2007/2016) *Acutely Ill Adults in Hospital: recognising and responding to deterioration*, NICE Clinical Guideline #CG50 [available at: https://www.nice.org.uk/guidance/CG50].

NICE (2014) *Developing NICE Guidelines: the manual* [available at: https://www.nice.org.uk/process/pmg20/chapter/introduction-and-overview].

Noble, H. and Smith, J. (2015) Issues of validity and reliability in qualitative research, *Evidence-Based Nursing*, 18 (2): 34–35.

Noyes, J. (2010) Never mind the qualitative, feel the depth! The evolving role of qualitative research in Cochrane intervention reviews, *Journal of Research in Nursing*, 15 (6): 525–534.

Nursing and Midwifery Council (NMC) (2015a) *Guidance on the Professional Duty of Candour: joint guidance with the General Medical Council on the duty of candour* [available at: https://www.nmc.org.uk/standards/guidance/the-professional-duty-of-candour/].

Nursing and Midwifery Council (NMC) (2015b) *The Code: Professional standards of practice and behaviour for nurses and midwives.* London: NMC [available at: https://www.nmc.org.uk/standards/code/].

Nursing and Midwifery Council (NMC) (2015c) *Raising Concerns: guidance for nurses and midwives* [available at: https://www.nmc.org.uk/standards/guidance/raising-concerns-guidance-for-nurses-and-midwives/].

Oldershaw, M. (2009) What are adult nursing students' attitudes towards patients with HIV/AIDS and what can be done to improve attitudes? Unpublished BSc

(Hons) dissertation, School of Health and Social Care, Oxford Brookes University, Oxford.

Parkhurst, J.O. and Abeysinghe, S. (2016) What constitutes 'good' evidence for public health and social policy-making? From hierarchies to appropriateness, *Social Epistemology*, 30 (5/6): 665–679.

Pauling, L. (1986) *How to Live Longer and Feel Better.* Corvallis, OR: Oregon State University Press.

Roever, L. (2015) Critical appraisal of a questionnaire study, *Evidence-Based Medicine and Practice*, 1: e110 [available at: https://www.omicsonline.org/open-access/critical-appraisal-of-a-questionnaire-study-ebmp-1000e110.php?aid=70356].

Rolls, K., Hansen, M., Jackson, D. and Elliott, D. (2016) How health care professionals use social media to create virtual communities: an integrative review, *Journal of Medical Internet Research*, 18 (6): e166.

Royal College of Nursing (RCN) (2014) *Good Practice for Handling Feedback* [available at: https://www.rcn.org.uk/professional-development/publications/pub-004725].

Ruth-Sahd, L. (2014) What lies within: phenomenology and intuitive self-knowledge, *Creative Nursing*, 20 (1): 21–29.

Rycroft-Malone, J., Seers, K., Chandler, J., Hawkes, C.A., Crichton, N., Allen, C. et al. (2013) The role of evidence, context, and facilitation in an implementation trial: implications for the development of the PARIHS framework, *Implementation Science*, 8 (1): 28.

Sackett, D.L., Rosenberg, W.M.C., Muir Gray, J.A., Haynes, R.B. and Richardson, W.S. (1996) Evidence based medicine: what it is and what it isn't, *British Medical Journal*, 312 (7023): 71–72.

Sackett, D.L., Straus, S.E., Richardson, W.S., Rosenburg, W. and Haynes, R.B. (2000) *Evidence-based Medicine: How to practise and teach EBM*, 2nd edn. London: Churchill Livingstone.

Scurlock-Evans, L., Upton, P. and Upton, D. (2014) Evidence-based practice in physiotherapy: a systematic review of barriers, enablers and interventions, *Physiotherapy*, 100 (3): 208–219.

Sharp, P. and Taylor, B. (2012) Prompt questions for randomised controlled trials and qualitative studies (unpublished). Oxford Brookes University.

Siering, U., Eikermann, M., Hausner, E., Hoffmann-Eßer, W. and Neugebauer, E.A. (2013) Appraisal tools for clinical practice guidelines: a systematic review, *PLoS One*, 8 (12): e82915 [available at: http://journals.plos.org/plosone/article?id=10.1371/journal.pone.0082915].

Sinclair, W., McLoughlin, M. and Warne, T. (2015) To twitter to woo: harnessing the power of social media (SoMe) in nurse education to enhance the student's experience, *Nurse Education in Practice*, 15 (6): 507–511.

Smith, J. and Judge, B. (2016) Effectiveness of the precordial thump in restoring heart rhythm following out-of-hospital cardiac arrest, *Emergency Medicine Journal*, 33 (5): 366–367.

Social Care Institute for Excellence (SCIE) (2016) *The Care Act: New opportunities for the voluntary, community and social enterprise sector.* SCIE Report #74. London: SCIE [available at: http://www.scie.org.uk/publications/reports/report74-care-act-and-vcse-sector.asp].

Souto, R.Q., Khanassov, V., Hong, Q.N., Bush, P.L., Vedel, I. and Pluye, P. (2015) Systematic mixed studies reviews: updating results on the reliability and efficiency of the mixed methods appraisal tool, *International Journal of Nursing Studies*, 52 (1): 500–501.

Squires, J., Sullivan, K., Eccles, M., Worswick, J. and Grimshaw, J. (2014) Are multifaceted interventions more effective than single-component interventions in changing health-care professionals' behaviours? An overview of systematic reviews, *Implementation Science*, 9: 152 [available at: http://implementation-science.biomedcentral.com/articles/10.1186/s13012-014-0152-6].

Sredl, D., Melnyk, B.M., Hsueh, K.-H., Jenkins, R., Ding, C. and Durham, J. (2011) Health care in crisis! Can nurse executives' beliefs about and implementation of evidence-based practice be key solutions in health care reform?, *Teaching and Learning in Nursing*, 6: 73–79.

Standing, M. (2005) Perceptions of clinical decision making skills on a developmental journey from student to staff nurse, PhD thesis, University of Kent, Canterbury.

Standing, M. (2014) *Clinical Judgement and Decision Making for Nursing Students*, 2nd edn. London: Learning Matters.

Standing, M. (2015) Patient assessment and decision making, in L. Howatson-Jones, M. Standing and S. Roberts, *Patient Assessment and Care Planning in Nursing*. London: Sage.

Stern, C., Jordan, Z. and McArthur, A. (2014) Developing the review question and inclusion criteria, *The American Journal of Nursing*, 114 (4): 53–56.

Stillwell, S.B., Fineout-Overholt, E., Melnyk, B.M. and Williamson, K.M. (2010) Asking the clinical question: a key step in evidence based practice, *American Journal of Nursing*, 110 (3): 58–61.

Sullivan, G., O'Brien, B. and Mwini-Nyaledzigbor, P. (2016) Sources of support for women experiencing obstetric fistula in northern Ghana: a focused ethnography, *Midwifery*, 40: 162–168.

Teng, A.M., Atkinson, J., Disney, G., Wilson, N. and Blakely, T. (2017) Changing socioeconomic inequalities in cancer incidence and mortality: cohort study with 54 million person-years follow up 1981–2011, *International Journal of Cancer*, 140 (6): 1306–1316.

Thompson, C., Aitken, L., Doran, D. and Dowding, D. (2013) An agenda for clinical decision making and judgement in nursing research and education, *International Journal of Nursing Studies*, 50 (12): 1720–1726.

Thompson, C. and Stapley, S. (2011) Do educational interventions improve nurses' clinical decision making and judgement? A systematic review, *International Journal of Nursing Studies*, 48 (7): 881–893.

Thouless, R.H. and Thouless, C.R. (1953) *Straight and Crooked Thinking*, 4th edn. Sevenoaks: Hodder & Stoughton.

Tiffen, J., Corbridge, S.J. and Slimmer, L. (2014) Enhancing clinical decision making: development of a contiguous definition and conceptual framework, *Journal of Professional Nursing*, 30 (5): 399–405.

Tilson, J.K., Kaplan, S.L., Harris, J.L., Hutchinson, A., Ilic, D., Niederman, R. et al. (2011) Sicily statement on classification and development of evidence-based practice learning assessment tools, *BMC Medical Education*, 11: 78 [available at: http://bmcmededuc.biomedcentral.com/articles/10.1186/1472-6920-11-78].

Titler, M.G., Conlon, P., Reynolds, M.A., Ripley, R., Tsodikov, A., Wilson, D.S. et al. (2016) The effect of a translating research into practice intervention to promote use of evidence-based fall prevention interventions in hospitalized adults: a prospective pre–post implementation study in the US, *Applied Nursing Research*, 31: 52–59.

Van Beek, K., Siouta, N., Preston, N., Hasselaar, J., Hughes, S., Payne, S. et al. (2016) To what degree is palliative care integrated in guidelines and pathways for adult cancer patients in Europe? a systematic literature review, *BMC Palliative Care*, 15: 26 [available at: http://bmcpalliatcare.biomedcentral.com/articles/10.1186/s12904-016-0100-0].

Van der Linden, S. (2016) Why doctors should convey the medical consensus on vaccine safety, *Evidence-Based Medicine*, 21 (3): 119.

Van El, C.G., Cornel, M.C., Borry, P., Hastings, R.J., Fellmann, F., Hodgson, S.V. et al. (2013) Whole-genome sequencing in health care, *European Journal of Human Genetics*, 21 (suppl. 1): S1–S5.

Van Zuuren, E.J., Fedorowicz, Z., Christensen, R., Lavrijsen, A. and Arents, B.W.M. (2017) Emollients and moisturisers for eczema, *Cochrane Database of Systematic Reviews*, 2: CD012119 [available at: http://onlinelibrary.wiley.com/doi/10.1002/14651858.CD012119.pub2/full].

Variend, H. (2012) Capacity confusion (letter), *British Medical Association News*, 1 September.

Viner, K. (2016) How technology disrupted the truth, *The Irish Times*, 11 July.

Wakefield, A.J., Murch, S.H., Anthony, A. and Linnell, J. (1998) Ileal-lymphoidnodular hyperplasia, non-specific colitis and pervasive developmental disorder in children, *Lancet*, 351: 637–641 [paper now withdrawn].

Warren, J.I., McLaughlin, M., Bardsley, J., Eich, J., Esche, C.A., Kropkowski, L. et al. (2016) The strengths and challenges of implementing EBP in healthcare systems, *Worldviews on Evidence-Based Nursing*, 13 (1): 15–24.

Watson, R. (2017) Beall's list of predatory open access journals: RIP, *Nursing Open*, 4 (2): 60.

Webster, J. and Osborne, S. (2015) Preoperative bathing or showering with skin antiseptics to prevent surgical site infection, *Cochrane Database of Systematic Reviews*, 2: CD004985 [available at: http://onlinelibrary.wiley.com/doi/10.1002/14651858.CD004985.pub5/full].

Williams, B., Brown, T. and Costello, S. (2015) A cross-cultural investigation into the dimensional structure and stability of the Barriers to Research and Utilization Scale (BARRIERS Scale), *BMC Research Notes*, 8: 601 [available at: https://bmcresnotes.biomedcentral.com/articles/10.1186/s13104-015-1579-9].

Wolfenden, L., Jones, J., Williams, C.M., Finch, M., Wyse, R.J., Kingsland, M. et al. (2016) Strategies to improve the implementation of healthy eating, physical activity and obesity prevention policies, practices or programmes within childcare services, *Cochrane Database of Systematic Reviews*, 10: CD011779 [available at: http://onlinelibrary.wiley.com/doi/10.1002/14651858.CD011779.pub2/full].

Wong, J.C., Levin, S. and Solon, O. (2016) Bursting the Facebook bubble: we asked voters on the left and right to swap feeds, *The Guardian*, 16 November [available at: https://www.theguardian.com/us-news/2016/nov/16/facebook-bias-bubble-us-election-conservative-liberal-news-feed].

Woodbury, M.G. and Kuhnke, J.L. (2014) Evidence-based vs. evidence-informed practice: What's the difference?, *Wound Care Canada*, 12 (1): 18–21.

World Medical Association (WMA) (2013) World Medical Association Declaration of Helsinki: ethical principles for medical research involving human subjects, *Journal of the American Medical Association*, 310 (20): 2191–2194.

Wright, K., Golder, S. and Lewis-Light, K. (2015) What value is the CINAHL database when searching for systematic reviews of qualitative studies?, *Systematic Reviews*, 4: 104 [available at: https://systematicreviewsjournal.biomedcentral. com/articles/10.1186/s13643-015-0069-4].

Yost, J., Ciliska, D. and Dobbins, M. (2014) Evaluating the impact of an intensive education workshop on evidence-informed decision making knowledge, skills, and behaviours: a mixed methods study, *BMC Medical Education*, 14: 13 [available at: http://bmcmededuc.biomedcentral.com/articles/10.1186/1472-6920-14-13].

Young, S., Adamou, M., Asherson, P., Coghill, D., Colley, B., Gudjonsson, G. et al. (2016) Recommendations for the transition of patients with ADHD from child to adult healthcare services: a consensus statement from the UK adult ADHD network, *BMC Psychiatry*, 16: 301 [available at: https://bmcpsychiatry.biomedcentral. com/articles/10.1186/s12888-016-1013-4].

Index

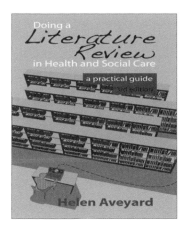

Doing a Literature Review in Health and Social Care
A Practical Guide
Third Edition

Helen Aveyard

9780335263073 (Paperback)
January 2014

eBook also available

This bestselling book is a step-by-step guide to doing a literature review in health and social care. It is vital reading for all those undertaking their undergraduate or postgraduate dissertation or any research module which involves a literature review. The book provides a practical guide to doing a literature review from start to finish.

Key features:

- Even more examples of real life research scenarios
- More emphasis on how to ask the right question
- New and updated advice on following a clear search strategy

www.openup.co.uk

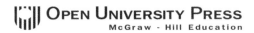 OPEN UNIVERSITY PRESS
McGraw - Hill Education

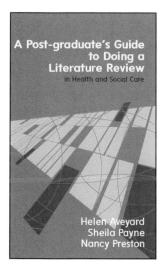

A Postgraduate's Guide to Doing a Literature Review in Health and Social Care

Helen Aveyard, Sheila Payne and Nancy Preston

9780335263684 (Paperback)
February 2016

eBook also available

This text is a comprehensive, highly readable guide to how to undertake a literature review in health and social care, tailored specifically for postgraduate study. Providing clarity and a step by step approach to doing a literature review from start to finish it will enable you to:

- Identify which type of review is appropriate for your study
- Select the literature that you need to include in your review
- Search for, appraise and analyse relevant literature
- Write up your review

The book explores the common features of a broad range of types of literature review, which serve different functions – including the literature review that is a pre-requisite prior to a larger empirical study, and the literature review that is a study in its own right. With real-life examples of written research and succinct summaries at the end of each chapter, this is the ideal text for students wanting to get the very most from their study.

www.openup.co.uk

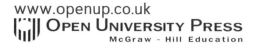

OPEN UNIVERSITY PRESS
McGraw - Hill Education